Minerals
Supplements
& Vitamins

THE ESSENTIAL GUIDE

Minerals
Supplements
& Vitamins

H. WINTER GRIFFITH, M.D.

Technical Consultant

Cynthia Thomson, Ph.D., R.D.

*Clinical Nutrition Research Specialist, Arizona Cancer Center
University of Arizona Prevention Center*

FISHER
BOOKS

Publishers: *Fred W. Fisher,*
  Helen V. Fisher & Howard W. Fisher
Managing Editor: *Sarah Trotta*
Editors: *Meg Morris, Melanie Mallon*
Consulting Editors: *Brian Engstrom,*
  Jean Anderson
Index: *Michelle B. Graye*
Production: *Randy Schultz, Ann Olsen*
Cover Photo: *Fisher Books Trannie*
Cover: *Gary D. Smith,*
  Performance Design

Published by Fisher Books, LLC
5225 W. Massingale Road
Tucson, Arizona 85743-8416
(520) 744-6110

Library of Congress
Cataloging-in-Publication Data

Griffith, H. Winter (Henry Winter), 1926-
  Minerals, supplements & vitamins : the
  essential guide / H. Winter Griffith ;
  technical adviser, Cynthia Thomson.
    p. cm.
  Includes bibliographical references
  and index.
  ISBN 1-55561-229-6
    1. Dietary supplements—Handbooks,
  manuals, etc. I. Title: Minerals,
  supplements, and vitamins. II. Thomson,
  Cynthia, 1957- III. Title.

RM217.2.G75 2000
613.2'85—dc21

                                    99-053244

Printed in U.S.A.
10 9 8 7 6 5 4 3 2 1

Contents

About the Author

H. Winter Griffith, M.D., received his medical degree from Emory University in 1953 and spent more than 20 years in private practice. At Florida State University, he established a basic medical science program and also directed the family practice residency program at Tallahassee Memorial Hospital. After moving to the Southwest, he became associate professor of Family and Community Medicine at the University of Arizona College of Medicine. He devoted most of his time to writing medical-information books for general readers.

Dedication

To each of you who wishes to be informed enough to become the most important member of your own healthcare team.

Acknowledgments

Several years ago, Dr. Griffith set a personal goal to translate complicated, technical medical information into easy-to-understand terms that anyone outside the healing professions could use. Four previous books dealing with medications, symptoms, surgery and sports injuries have been major steps toward that goal.

Dr. Griffith remained a student of medicine for 40 years. The need for this book was made clear during his experience as a family doctor, teacher and author, answering questions (or seeking answers) for patients, medical students, nurses and physicians in training.

Special thanks to Sheldon Saul Hendler, M.D., Ph.D., author of *The Complete Guide to the Anti-Aging Nutrients* (Simon & Schuster, 1984; Fireside, 1986) for allowing the use of his material and unique research insights in this book.

Thanks also to everyone else who helped with this book in so many ways, including Brian Engstrom and Jean Anderson, research assistants, and technical consultant Cynthia Thomson, Ph.D., R.D., who is a registered dietitian with more than 18 years of clinical experience in nutrition. She recently completed her Ph.D. in Nutritional Sciences at the University of Arizona, where she also works as an investigator on nutritional breast-cancer research trials. She facilitates the Nutritional Medicine Core for the Department of Medicine's program in Integrative Medicine, the first such training program in the United States.

Last but not least, thanks to the authors and publishers of the reference material (listed in the Bibliography) that was so helpful in the preparation of this book.

Minerals and Vitamins

With the increased popularity of dietary supplements come questions regarding truthfulness in advertising and product safety. As with food, federal law requires manufacturers of dietary supplements to ensure that the products they put on the market are safe. But supplement manufacturers do not have to provide information to the Food and Drug Administration (FDA) to get a product on the market, unlike the food additive process often required of new food ingredients. FDA review and approval of supplement ingredients and products is not required before marketing.

Claims that tout a supplement's healthful benefits have always been a controversial feature of dietary supplements. Manufacturers often rely on them to sell their products, but consumers wonder if they can trust these claims. Under the Dietary Supplement and Health Education Act (DSHEA) of 1994, manufacturers are allowed to use three types of claims: nutrient content claims, disease claims and nutrition support claims.

Nutrient content claims describe the level of a particular nutrient in a food or dietary supplement. For example, a supplement containing at least 200 milligrams of calcium per serving could carry the claim "high in calcium." A supplement with at least 12 milligrams per serving of vitamin C could state on its label, "Excellent source of vitamin C."

Disease claims show a link between a food or substance and a disease or health-related condition. FDA authorizes these claims based on a review of the scientific evidence.

Nutrition support claims can describe a link between a nutrient and the deficiency disease that can result if the nutrient is lacking in the diet. For example, the label of a vitamin C supplement could state that vitamin C prevents scurvy. When these types of claims are used, the label must mention the prevalence of the nutrient deficiency disease in the United States.

Even with increased FDA scrutiny, consumers and manufacturers, not the government, are responsible for checking the safety of dietary supplements and determining the truthfulness of label claims.

Effective in March 1999, the following information must appear on the labels of dietary supplements:

- Statement of identity (for example, "acidophilus")
- Net quantity of contents (for example, "60 capsules")
- Structure-function claim *and* the message "This statement has not been evaluated by the Food and Drug Administration. This product is not intended to diagnose, treat, cure or prevent any disease." (A structure-function claim refers to the purpose of or benefit derived from using the product.)
- Directions for use (for example, "Take one capsule daily.")
- Supplement Facts Panel (lists serving size, amount and active ingredient)
- Other ingredients in descending order of predominance and by common name or proprietary blend
- Name and place of business of manufacturer, packer or distributor (This is the address to which to write for more product information)

In addition, the American Institute of Nutrition and the American Society for Clinical Nutrition have issued an official statement on vitamin and mineral supplements. This statement was developed jointly with the American Dietetic Association and the National Council against Health Fraud. The American Medical Association's Council on Scientific Affairs reviewed the statement and found it to be consistent with its official statement on dietary supplements.

The statement reads: "Healthy children and adults should obtain adequate nutrient intakes from dietary sources. Meeting nutrient needs by choosing a variety of foods in moderation, rather than by supplementation, reduces the potential risk for both nutrient deficiencies and nutrient excesses. Individual recommendations regarding supplements and diets should come from physicians and registered dietitians."

Supplementation is sometimes necessary in various circumstances. Some of these situations are listed below.

- Women with excessive menstrual bleeding may need iron supplements.
- Pregnant or breastfeeding women have an increased need for certain nutrients, especially iron, folic acid and calcium.
- People with very low calorie intakes frequently consume diets that do not meet their needs for most nutrients.
- Some vegetarians may not receive adequate calcium, iron, zinc and vitamin B-12.
- Newborns are commonly given a single dose of vitamin K to prevent abnormal bleeding. (This is done under the direction of a physician.)
- Certain disorders or diseases and some medications interfere with nutrient intake, digestion, absorption, metabolism or excretion. In addition, expanding scientific

research indicates that supplementation with specific nutrients may help prevent disease. Those who suffer myocardial infarction, for example, may benefit from vitamin-E supplementation.

Nutrients are potentially toxic when ingested in sufficiently large amounts. Safe intake levels vary widely from nutrient to nutrient and may vary with an individual's age and health. In addition, high-dosage vitamin and mineral supplements can interfere with the normal metabolism of other nutrients and with the therapeutic effects of certain drugs. The Recommended Dietary Allowance (RDA) and the Dietary Reference Intake (DRI) represent the best currently available assessments of safe and adequate intakes. They serve as the basis for the Recommended Daily Allowances shown on many product labels, although these are determined by the FDA for labeling purposes and should not be used by individuals as guidelines for their own daily intake. *Recommended Daily Allowances are not the same as Recommended Dietary Allowances.*

Every health professional wants consumers to take proper nutrients and supplements if they need them, but some people abuse these essential substances by taking doses 10 to 20 times the recommended amount or more.

Some people believe if one pill is good, 20 pills must be better. They also believe minerals, supplements and vitamins are medicine.

As information in this book points out, minerals, supplements and vitamins can cause side effects, adverse reactions and interactions with other drugs and nutrients. Many individuals need to avoid certain substances because of a unique situation, such as pregnancy or age. Others need to be aware that medical conditions, such as heart problems or various disease conditions, can be an indication not to take certain substances.

When deciding whether or not to supplement your diet with minerals and vitamins, remember that too much can be harmful. For example, high doses of vitamin A can cause bone pain and vomiting. High doses of vitamin C can also have toxic effects, including diarrhea and perhaps kidney stones. Too much of this vitamin can interfere with white blood cells' ability to kill bacteria. This can make infections worse rather than clear them up.

Many conditions may also rule out taking some substances. Always be alert to any side effects or interactions you may experience that could put your health in jeopardy. It's up to you to be a "smart" consumer of the minerals, supplements and vitamins your body may need. Get them from the food you eat when you can—supplement with available products when you must.

Minerals

Minerals are inorganic chemical elements. They participate in many biochemical and physiological processes necessary for optimum growth, development and health. There is a clear and important distinction between the terms *mineral* and *trace element*. If the body requires more than 100 milligrams of a mineral each day, the substance is labeled *mineral.* If the body requires less than 100 milligrams of a mineral each day, the substance is labeled *trace element.*

Many minerals are essential parts of enzymes. They also participate actively in regulating many physiological functions, including transporting oxygen to each of the body's 60 trillion cells, providing the stimulus for muscles to contract and in many ways guaranteeing normal function of the central nervous system. Minerals are required for growth, maintenance, repair and health of tissues and bones.

Most minerals are widely distributed in foods. *Severe mineral deficiency is unusual in the Western world.* Of all essential minerals, only a few may be deficient in a typical diet. Iron deficiency can be seen in infants, children and pregnant women. Zinc and copper deficiencies are also not uncommon, especially during illness.

Vitamins

Vitamins are chemical compounds necessary for growth, health, normal metabolism and physical well-being. Some vitamins are essential parts of *enzymes*—the chemical molecules that catalyze or facilitate the completion of chemical reactions. Other vitamins form essential parts of *hormones*—the chemical substances that promote and protect body health and reproduction. If you're in good health, you need vitamins only in small amounts. They can be found in sufficient quantities in the foods you eat, assuming you eat a normal, well-balanced diet of foods grown in nutritionally adequate soil.

Traditionally, vitamins have been divided into two categories: *fat-soluble* and *water-soluble.*

Fat-soluble vitamins can be stored in the body. If you take excessive amounts of fat-soluble vitamins, they accumulate to provide needed amounts at a later time. That's the good news. The bad news is, if you take excessive amounts of fat-soluble vitamins, toxic levels can accumulate in storage areas such as the liver. Too much of any fat-soluble vitamin can lead to potentially dangerous, long-term physical problems.

Water-soluble vitamins cannot be stored in the body to any great extent. The daily amount you need must be provided by what you eat over several days.

The amount of vitamins you need increases during illness, following surgery or even as a result of the aging process. In these circumstances, vitamin supplements may be necessary to meet increased needs or prevent a deficiency of select nutrients. People with special needs for supplements or others at risk of vitamin deficiency are identified and discussed in detail later in this section (see page 10).

Vitamin supplements cannot take the place of good nutrition. Vitamins do not provide energy. Your body needs other substances besides vitamins for adequate nutrition, including carbohydrates, fats, proteins and minerals. Vitamins cannot help maintain a healthy body except in the presence of other nutrients, mainly from food and minerals.

Multivitamin/Mineral Preparations

A varied diet will contain all the nutrients you need. For healthy people food is the best, most reliable source of nutrients. If you or your children need supplementation, the best place to start is by taking one of the commercially available multivitamin/mineral preparations. Commercial over-the-counter products usually have a good balance of nutrients. Taking separate products can lead to an imbalance of nutrients, which can lead to an overabundance of one substance at the expense of decreased absorption or effectiveness of another.

Taking separate, individual nutrient supplements will require careful consideration of nutrient-to-nutrient interactions and is more likely to result in excess intake above what may be healthy—in these cases you may want to talk with your doctor, dietitian or pharmacist. The cost tends to be lower if you take a combination product rather than separate products.

Most major pharmaceutical manufacturers supply widely advertised combination products. The brand names are too numerous to list and they change constantly. Your pharmacist, doctor or dietitian should be able to recommend a good source for a superior multivitamin/mineral preparation.

If you study minerals and vitamins, you may find you need supplements for one reason or another. We hope this book provides you with enough information to choose wisely or be able to ask the right questions to find out what is best for you.

Guide to Mineral, Vitamin and Acid Charts

Information in this book is organized in condensed, easy-to-read charts, divided into four main sections: minerals, amino acids and nucleic acids, supplements and vitamins. (Information on the supplement charts begins on page 18.) Each substance is described in a multi-page format as shown in the sample charts on the following pages. They are arranged alphabetically by the most frequently recognized name—usually a generic name instead of a brand name.

The most common names of substances appear at the top of the chart. For example, vitamin C is frequently called *ascorbic acid.* Both names appear at the top of the chart. Less common names are listed in the first section of the chart, *Basic Information.*

To learn more about any mineral or vitamin, you need to know only one name. Look in the Index (page 196) for any name you know. The Index provides a page number for the information you seek about that substance.

The next few pages provide an explanation for each section of a mineral, vitamin or acid chart. The numbers correspond to the sample chart on pages 8 and 9. This information will help you read and understand the charts that begin on page 25.

1–Generic name

Each chart is titled by the *generic name,* the official chemical name of the substance. If two or more generic names exist, the substance is alphabetized by the most common name, with other names in parentheses at the top of the page or listed under the *Basic Information* section. If a substance has two or more generic names, the Index includes a reference for each name.

A product container may show a generic name, a brand name or both. If the container has no name, ask the pharmacist or health-store attendant for the name.

2–Available from natural sources?

3–Available from synthetic sources?

Many minerals, vitamins and supplements are advertised as

6

"natural," implying the product is derived from natural sources as opposed to synthetic sources. By definition, minerals are basic chemical substances that can't be manufactured (or synthesized) from other substances. However, many vitamins and supplements are derived from both natural and synthetic sources.

This is confusing to many consumers. Many manufacturers have done everything possible to take financial advantage of that confusion. Advertisers claim natural sources are good and synthetic sources are bad. The truth is, natural and synthetic versions of the same chemical are identical!

Don't pay extra money for *natural* vitamins or supplements. They all have the same effect on your body. The *synthetic* version may be even purer or less contaminated with extraneous materials such as insecticides and fertilizers.

4–Prescription required?

Most minerals, supplements and vitamins are available without prescription. Some formulas with higher dosages to treat specific diseases require a prescription from your doctor. "Yes" means your doctor must prescribe. "No" means you can buy this product without prescription. "Yes, for some" means that certain dosages or forms (such as an injection) require a prescription while others do not.

The information about a generic product is the same, whether it requires a prescription or not. If the generic ingredients are the same, nonprescription products have the same uses, dangers, warnings, precautions, side effects and interactions with other substances that prescription products do.

5–Fat-soluble or water-soluble?

This line applies *only* to vitamins. Fat-soluble vitamins can accumulate in the body and might cause toxic effects in excessive doses, either in a single day or in small, periodic excesses over a long time. Water-soluble vitamins do not accumulate to any great extent in the body. Except under unusual circumstances, the body readily eliminates excess water-soluble accumulation. The dangers of water-soluble vitamins generally depend on the effects of excessive dosages taken over a relatively short period.

6–Optimal Intake information

This line points you to the page where you'll find information about the substance's Daily Value, Recommended Dietary Allowance (RDA), Dietary Reference Intake (DRI), Tolerable Upper Intake and Optimal Intake whenever this information is available. Not all substances will have this information for a few possible reasons: Some substances are still under study;

Sample Chart

1 ———— ## Pantothenic Acid (Vitamin B-5)

Basic Information

2 ————
3 ————
4 ————
5
6 ————

- Available from natural sources? Yes
- Available from synthetic sources? Yes
- Prescription required? No
- Water-soluble
- *Optimal Intake*, see pages 182–183

7 ———— ### Natural Sources

Avocados   Meats, all kinds
Bananas   Milk
Blue cheese   Oranges
Broccoli   Peanut butter
Chicken   Peanuts
Collard greens   Peas
Eggs   Soybeans
Lentils   Sunflower seeds
Liver   Wheat germ
Lobster   Whole-grain products

8 ———— ### Benefits

- Promotes normal growth and development
- Aids release of energy from foods
- Helps synthesize numerous body materials

9 ———— ### Possible Additional Benefits

- May stimulate wound healing in animals
- May alleviate stress
- May reduce fatigue

Who May Benefit from Additional Amounts? ———— 10

- Anyone with inadequate caloric or nutritional dietary intake or increased nutritional requirements
- People more than 55 years old with vitamin-B deficiencies
- Pregnant or breastfeeding women
- Those who abuse alcohol or other drugs
- People with a chronic wasting illness, including sprue, celiac disease, regional enteritis
- Those under excess stress for long periods
- Anyone who has recently undergone surgery
- Athletes and workers who participate in vigorous physical activities

VITAMINS

Deficiency Symptoms ———— 11

No proven symptoms exist for pantothenic acid alone. However, lack of one B vitamin usually means lack of other B nutrients. Pantothenic acid is usually given with other B vitamins if there are symptoms of any vitamin-B deficiency, including excessive fatigue, sleep disturbances, loss of appetite, nausea or dermatitis.

Usage Information

What this vitamin does: ———— 12
Vitamin B-5 is converted to a coenzyme (see Glossary) in energy metabolism of carbohydrates, protein and fat.

———— 13

➤

108   PANTOTHENIC ACID

14

Available as:
• Tablets: Swallow whole with a full glass of liquid. Don't chew or crush. Take with or 1 to 1-1/2 hours after meals unless otherwise directed by your doctor.
• Vitamin B-5 is a constituent of many multivitamin/mineral preparations and B-complex vitamins.

15

Warnings and Precautions

Don't take if you are:
• Allergic to pantothenic acid
• Taking levodopa for Parkinson's disease

16

Consult your doctor if you have: Hemophilia.

17

Over 55:
No problems are expected.

18

Pregnancy:
Don't exceed recommended dose.

19

Breastfeeding:
Don't exceed recommended dose.

20

Effect on lab tests:
No expected effects.

21

Storage:
• Store in a cool, dry place away from direct light, but don't freeze.
• Store safely out of reach of children.
• Don't store in bathroom medicine cabinet. Heat and moisture may change the action of the vitamin.

22

Others:
Avoid doses greater than five times the DRI.

23
24

Overdose/Toxicity

What to do:

For symptoms of overdose:
Discontinue vitamin and consult doctor. Also see *Adverse Reactions or Side Effects* section below.

For accidental overdose (such as child taking entire bottle): Dial 911 (emergency), 0 for operator or call your nearest Poison Control Center.

Adverse Reactions or Side Effects — **25**

Reaction or effect	What to do
Diarrhea	Discontinue or reduce close to DRI levels.

Interaction with Medicine, Minerals or Vitamins — **26**

Interacts with	Combined effect
Levodopa	Small amounts of pantothenic acid nullify levodopa's effect. Carbidopa-levodopa combination is not affected by this interaction.

Interaction with Other Substances — **27**

Tobacco decreases absorption. Smokers may require supplemental pantothenic acid.

Lab Tests to Detect Deficiency — **28**

Methods are limited and expensive. Tests are used only for research at present. Methods are available to measure blood levels and levels in 24-hour urine collections.

some substances are abundantly available in food, so deficiency and excess are rare to non-existent and no guidelines are necessary; some substances are so rare, no guidelines have been established.

7–Natural Sources

This section lists the food and beverage sources from which minerals, vitamins and acids may be obtained. They are listed alphabetically, not in order of the richest sources of the substance. If you want more information about natural sources, many reference works are available at your local library.

8–Benefits

This section consists of *proved benefits,* including body functions the substance maintains or improves. It also lists disease processes and malfunctions the substance cures or improves. These proved benefits have withstood the scrutiny of scientifically controlled studies with results published in medical literature. This medical literature is subjected to review by top authorities in many fields before the material can be published in respected scientific journals.

9–Possible Additional Benefits

Some authors and many newspaper, magazine and television advertisers make unjustified, sometimes outrageous, claims for products. This list contains claims that have *not* withstood the same scientific scrutiny the *Benefits* section has passed. These claims may be as accurate and as effective as the proven claims, but they haven't been proved with well-controlled studies. Such studies can take years to complete and may be very expensive. Until such studies have been completed, the claims must be listed as possible additional benefits. Do not self-medicate based on these unproven benefits!

10–Who May Benefit from Additional Amounts?

People listed in this category are most likely to need significant care to regain or maintain normal health or are less likely to meet their requirements through diet alone. A summary of groups follows, with a list of reasons why the risk is greater.

Anyone with inadequate dietary intake or increased nutritional needs—Included in this group are people whose energy needs are less than 1,200 calories a day. Fewer than 1,200 calories a day for energy requirements almost never provides enough minerals and vitamins, so supplements are needed. Those most likely to have inadequate dietary intake include

- People of small stature or build who eat only minimal nutrients per day to maintain current weight
- Elderly people with greatly decreased daily activities, particularly aging women

❧ People who have had limbs amputated

❧ People with reduced physical activity because of activity-limiting disease, such as coronary-artery disease, intermittent lameness, angina pectoris

❧ Fad dieters with a dietary imbalance and inadequacy

❧ People with eating disorders such as anorexia nervosa or bulimia

❧ Vegetarians

People over 55—People in this age group may have inadequate dietary intake because of difficulty obtaining an adequate diet, or because of disability and depression.

Pregnancy—Pregnant women uniformly need supplementation of folic acid and iron. Sometimes they need other supplements as well. Pregnant women need to increase dietary intake so total body weight increases from 12 to 30 pounds during pregnancy. Many women do not consume enough calories to allow this weight gain and therefore develop a nutritional deficiency. This causes a need for supplementation with a well-rounded, well-balanced preparation containing minerals and vitamins in addition to separate supplementation of folic acid and iron.

Ask your doctor to recommend specific brand names of acceptable multivitamin/mineral preparations. Also seek advice about folic acid and iron.

Breastfeeding women—Breastfeeding women who are healthy and active may need to continue supplementation, especially iron. Consult your doctor.

Most authorities suggest that iron and folic-acid supplements for pregnant and breastfeeding women should be taken as separate products. Iron occasionally causes gastrointestinal side effects that are so uncomfortable to some women that they discontinue the supplements.

Another important nutritional factor with breastfeeding is the need for extra fluids. Fluid deficiency can be as disabling as a nutritional deficiency. Drink at least eight 8-ounce glasses of water a day.

People who abuse alcohol and other drugs—People who consume too much alcohol are likely to develop nutritional deficiencies. Much of the daily caloric intake of these people is the alcohol they consume, which is deficient in nutritional substances. In addition, alcohol abusers have poor food absorption and increased excretion of nutrients because of diarrhea and fluid loss. When the excessive alcohol consumption stops, the nutritional deficiency can be treated with good food and supplements for a while, if liver disease has not already occurred.

Abuse of other drugs frequently leads to decreased appetite and decreased interest in food. Addicts need supplements of both minerals and vitamins.

People with a chronic wasting illness—This group includes people with malignant disease, chronic malabsorption, hyperthyroidism, chronic obstructive pulmonary disease, congestive heart failure, cystic fibrosis and other illnesses. Nutritional risk is increased because these people have greatly increased caloric and nutritional requirements that are difficult to satisfy with food.

People who have recently undergone surgery—Surgery can cause a relative deficiency, even if a person is well nourished before surgery. People who have undergone surgery on the gastrointestinal tract are particularly likely to develop deficiencies during the post-operative period. Supplementation is very helpful. Minerals and vitamins are frequently administered intravenously until the patient can eat. After that, most people benefit from vitamin and mineral supplements for several weeks after the operation.

People with a portion of the gastrointestinal tract removed—These people are likely to develop deficiencies because important nutrient-absorbing parts of the gastrointestinal tract may be absent from the body. A good multivitamin/ mineral preparation usually prevents signs and symptoms of deficiencies. People who have had a significant portion of the stomach removed must take Vitamin B-12 supplements for life (usually by injection).

People who must take medicines—Many medications can cause a deficiency of minerals and vitamins. Specific drugs are listed in the *Interaction with Medicine, Minerals or Vitamins* section of each chart. For example, laxatives, antacids, medicines to treat epilepsy and oral contraceptives are a few of the medications that can cause a special need for supplementation of certain minerals and vitamins.

People with recent severe burns or injuries—The nutritional requirements for these people are greatly increased. Adequate supplementation can speed healing and recovery. Ask your doctor for specific advice.

11–Deficiency Symptoms

This section contains a list of proven symptoms of deficiency that have withstood the scrutiny of scientifically controlled studies with results published in medical literature.

12–What this substance does

This section includes a brief discussion of the part each substance plays in chemical reactions or combinations that affect growth, development and health maintenance.

13–Miscellaneous information

Information in this section doesn't fit readily into other information blocks on the charts. For example:

- Cooking tips to preserve the substance during food preparation

❧ Time lapse before changes can be expected

❧ Information of special interest

If no miscellaneous information exists for a particular substance, this section will be missing (as it is in the sample chart).

14–Available as

Minerals, vitamins and acids are often available in different forms. These include injections, tablets, powders, capsules and other oral forms.

15–Don't take if you

This section lists circumstances when use of this mineral, vitamin or acid may not be safe. In formal medical literature, these circumstances are called *absolute contraindications.* If no contraindications exist, this section will be missing.

16–Consult your doctor if you

This section lists conditions under which a mineral, vitamin or acid should be used with caution. In formal medical literature, these circumstances are frequently listed as *relative contraindications.* Using this product under these circumstances may require special consideration on your part and your doctor's. The guiding rule: *The potential benefit must outweigh the possible risk!* If no relative contraindications exist, this section will be missing.

17–Over 55

As a person ages, physical changes occur that require special consideration when using minerals, vitamins and acids. Liver and kidney functions usually decrease, metabolism slows and other changes take place. These are expected and must be considered.

Most chemical substances introduced into the body are metabolized or excreted at a rate that depends on kidney and liver functions. In the aging population, smaller doses or longer intervals between doses may be necessary to prevent an unhealthy concentration of minerals, vitamins or acids. These principles are exactly the same for therapeutic medicines and drugs. Toxic effects, severe side effects and adverse reactions occur more frequently and may cause more serious problems in this age group. If no special considerations exist, this section will be missing.

18–Pregnancy

Pregnancy creates an increased need for optimal nutrition, which may be difficult to maintain without using some supplemental minerals and vitamins. What you take depends on your age, your present state of nutrition, your state of health and other factors. Work with your doctor to determine what supplements you will need and how much. Don't take any substance without consulting your doctor first!

19–Breastfeeding

Lactating mothers require sound nutrition. Follow your doctor's recommendations about diet, minerals and vitamins during this time. Don't be reluctant to ask questions and challenge your doctor regarding these important topics. But don't take any substance without consulting your doctor first!

20–Effect on lab tests

This section lists lab studies that may be affected when you take minerals, supplements or vitamins. Possible effects include causing a false-positive or false-negative test, resulting in a low result or high result when your actual physical state is the opposite. In general, some tests can be performed accurately only after discontinuing minerals, vitamins or acids for a few days before the test is scheduled. If no effects are known, this section will be missing.

21–Storage

This section discusses how and where to store minerals, vitamins and acids, with an important reminder: Always store safely away from children!

22–Others

Special warnings and precautions appear here if they don't fit in any other specific information block. This section may contain information about the best time to take the substance, instructions about mixing or diluting or anything else that is important about this substance. If no additional warnings or precautions exist for a particular substance, this section will be missing, as it is in the sample chart.

23–Signs and symptoms

Symptoms listed here are the ones most likely to develop with toxicity or accidental or deliberate overdose. An overdosed person may not show all symptoms listed and may experience other symptoms not listed. Sometimes signs and symptoms are identical with ones listed as side effects or adverse reactions. The difference is intensity and severity. You must be the judge. Consult a doctor or poison control center if you are in doubt. If no signs or symptoms exist, this section will be missing, as it is in the sample chart.

24–What to do

If you suspect an overdose or toxicity, whether symptoms are apparent or not, follow instructions in this section. Expanded instructions for *anaphylaxis*— a severe, life-threatening allergic reaction—appear in the Glossary, page 186.

25–Adverse Reactions or Side Effects

Adverse reactions or side effects are symptoms that may occur when you ingest any substance, whether it is food, medicine, mineral, supplement or vitamin. These are effects on the body other than the desired effect for which you take them.

The term *side effect* may include an expected, perhaps unavoidable, effect of a mineral, vitamin or acid. For example, various forms of niacin may cause dramatic dizziness and flushing of the face and neck in the blush zone in almost everyone who takes a high enough dose. These symptoms are harmless, although sometimes uncomfortable, and have nothing to do with the intended use or therapeutic effect of niacin.

The term *adverse reaction* is more significant. These reactions can cause hazards that outweigh benefits. The "What to do" column will tell you what to do for each reaction listed.

26–Interaction with Medicine, Minerals or Vitamins

Minerals, supplements, vitamins and various medicines may interact in your body with other minerals, supplements, vitamins and medicines. It doesn't matter if they are prescription or nonprescription, natural or synthetic. Interactions affect absorption, elimination or distribution of the substances that interact with each other. Sometimes the interaction is beneficial, but at other times deadly. You may not be able to determine from the chart whether an interaction is good or bad. Don't guess! Ask your doctor or pharmacist—some interactions can kill!

27–Interaction with Other Substances

This list includes possible interactions with food, beverages, tobacco, cocaine, alcohol and other substances you may ingest.

If this section is missing, no known sigificant interactions exist.

28–Lab Tests to Detect Deficiency

Sometimes clinical features— medical history, signs and symptoms as interpreted by a competent professional—are all that are required to make an accurate diagnosis of deficiency. At other times, although clinical features may suggest a specific diagnosis, objective proof by a specific laboratory test adds confidence. As much data as can be collected is desirable before committing to a prolonged, sometimes expensive, sometimes hazardous course of treatment. When lab tests are readily available and reasonable in cost, doctors can treat their patients with greater confidence than is possible without laboratory confirmation of the diagnosis. This section lists many of those studies.

Note: Analysis of hair samples to detect deficiencies of minerals and trace elements, while easily available commercially, cannot be regarded as a valid test. Minerals and trace elements appear in shampoos, hair-care products and generally in the environment. In addition, when nutrition is poor for any reason, hair growth actually slows—causing greater concentration of minerals in the hair. This greater concentration gives falsely high values. Hair tests are entirely without value except for experimental purposes.

Supplements

Supplements are chemical substances that are neither minerals nor vitamins, but they have received notice as nutritional supplements. Many supplements have proven effects in the body but may not yet have proved safe and effective when taken in pill or capsule form to supplement normal food intake. Speculated benefits and claims frequently go beyond what can be proved at present. These include antiaging properties and claims that substances create and preserve health.

People separate into two distinct groups almost immediately when talk turns to supplementation. On one hand, the traditional medical establishment usually cries, "Eat a well-balanced diet, and you will get all the carbohydrates, fat, fiber, protein, minerals, vitamins and micronutrients you need." But hard data now available about our "normal, well-balanced" diet shows we are overfed and undernourished. The majority of experts in the medical field and in nutrition now agree: We consume too many calories, too much fat, too little fiber, too much refined sugar, too much sodium and not enough unrefined carbohydrates, making it difficult to maximize our health through diet.

On the other hand, some view every new supplement or every new promising piece of information about the existing supplements as a miracle that will cure our ills if the overly conservative medical establishment and the FDA will get out of the way. Advertisers are quite successful with this group because many people are easily persuaded that if they take a product, they will be healthier, live longer and look and feel sexier, slimmer and smarter.

Not much is written that takes a middle ground, even though this position probably represents the true status of human nutrition at present. This book *does* take a middle ground! It does not express any personal opinion—only the consensus of the majority of experts, presented as impartially as possible.

Labeling

Currently, supplements are regulated under the Dietary Supplement Act of 1994. This act states that supplement labels can only display information related to the structure and function of the supplement and not directly link it to prevention or treatment of disease. The burden of proving false claims or harm remains with the FDA.

In 1998, the FDA Modernization Act of 1997 took effect. According to this law, manufacturers are now permitted to use claims if such claims are based on current, published, authoritative statements from the National Institutes of Health (NIH), Center for Disease Control and Prevention (CDC), the Surgeon General, the Food and Safety Inspection Service and the Agricultural Research Service within the Department of Agriculture.

Guide to Supplement Charts

The food supplement information in this book is organized into condensed, easy-to-read charts. Each supplement is described on a 1- to 2-page chart, as shown in the sample chart opposite. Charts are arranged alphabetically by the most common name. If you cannot find a name, look for alternative names in the Index or ask your health-product retailer for alternative names.

A–Popular name

Each chart is titled by the most popular name. When there is more than one popular name, alternative names are shown in parentheses. If a supplement has several possible names, you'll find the least common listed under *Basic Information*. The Index contains a reference to each name listed. Popular names may vary in different parts of the world.

B–Chemicals this supplement contains

Chemicals and family names of chemically related groups are listed in this section.

C–Known Effects

This section lists identified chemical actions of the medicinal herb or supplement being discussed. These effects have been identified and validated by scientists and researchers through various studies. Some effects may be beneficial; others are harmful.

D–Miscellaneous information

This section contains information that doesn't fit into other information blocks on the chart. If no additional information exists, this section will be missing.

E–Possible Additional Effects

This list contains symptoms or medical problems this drug has been *reported* to treat or improve. These claims may be accurate, but they haven't been proved with well-controlled studies.

Sample Chart

146 ACIDOPHILUS

A — ## Acidophilus (Lactobacillus)

Basic Information

Acidophilus is a bacterium found in yogurt, kefir and other products.

B — Chemical this supplement contains: enzymes to aid digestion

Known Effects

C —

• Helps maintain normal bacteria balance in lower intestines
• Kills monilia, yeast and fungus on contact

D — **Miscellaneous information:**
Acidophilus is made by fermenting milk using *lactobacillus acidophilus* and other bacteria.

E — ### Possible Additional Effects

• May lower cholesterol
• May clear up skin problems
• May help prevent vaginal yeast infections in women who take antibiotics or who have diabetes
• May extend life span
• Potential aid for digestion of milk and milk products in people with lactase deficiency
• May enhance immunity
• May reduce symptoms from spastic colon
• May reduce diarrhea related to long-term antibiotic use
• May reduce diarrhea related to chemotherapy or radiation therapy

Warnings and Precautions

F — **Don't take if you:**
• Have intestinal problems, except under medical supervision
• Plan to use in vaginal area for yeast infections

Consult your doctor if you: — **G**
Take any medicinal drugs or herbs including aspirin, laxatives, cold and cough remedies, antacids, vitamins, minerals, amino acids, supplements, other prescription or nonprescription drugs.

Pregnancy: — **H**
Problems in pregnant women taking small or usual amounts have not been proved, but the chance of problems does exist. Don't use unless prescribed by your doctor.

Breastfeeding: — **I**
Problems in breastfed infants of lactating mothers taking small or usual amounts have not been proved, but the chance of problems does exist. Don't use unless prescribed by your doctor.

Infants and children: — **J**
Treating infants and children under 2 with any supplement is hazardous.

Others: — **K**
No problems expected if you are not pregnant and do not take amounts larger than the manufactirer's recommended dosage.

Storage: — **L**
• Store in cool, dry place away from direct light, but don't freeze.
• Store safely out of reach of children.
• Don't store in bathroom medicine cabinet. Heat and moisture may change the action of the supplement.

Safe dosage: — **M**
• At present no "safe" dosage has been established.
• It is available as a liquid, in capsules or tablets, as a powder or in milk products, such as yogurt or kefir.

Toxicity — **N**
Comparative-toxicity rating is not available from standard references.

Adverse Reactions, Side Effects or Overdose Symptoms — **O**
None are expected.

F–Don't take if you

Here you'll find circumstances under which the use of this supplement may not be safe. In formal medical literature, these circumstances are listed as *absolute contraindications.*

G–Consult your doctor if you

This section lists conditions in which this supplement should be used with caution. In formal medical literature, these circumstances are called *relative contraindications.* Using a supplement under these circumstances may require special consideration by you and your doctor. The guiding rule: *The potential benefit must outweigh the possible risk!*

H–Pregnancy

The more we learn about effective medications, the more healthcare workers fear the possible effects of any medicinal product on an unborn child. This fear holds for *all* chemicals that cause changes in the body. *The best rule to follow is don't take anything during pregnancy if you can avoid it!*

I–Breastfeeding

Although a breastfeeding infant is not as likely to be harmed as an unborn fetus, be cautious. If you take a medicine or a supplement during the time you breastfeed, do so *only* under professional supervision.

J–Infants and children

Treating infants and children under 2 years old with any supplement is hazardous. Dosages, uses and effects of a supplement cannot be gauged easily with a young child. Do not use supplements to treat a problem your child may have without first discussing it thoroughly with your doctor.

K–Others

Warnings and precautions appear here if they don't fit into other categories.

L–Storage

This section advises you on how to store supplements to best preserve them. It also includes a crucial reminder: *Always store any supplement safely away from children!*

M–Safe dosage

Safe dosages of many supplements have not been documented by procedures outlined by the FDA. For these, it is impossible to list a "safe" dosage and have it carry any significance. People who have had experience with supplements are usually qualified to predict safe doses if they know the person's age, medical history and some important facts about his or her current health.

Many reputable distributors of supplements have recommendations for ranges of safety, but these may vary a great deal from manufacturer to manufacturer, according to age and purity of the product. The most important fact to understand is the more you ingest over a long period of time, the more likely a toxic reaction will occur. Most available supplements are safe when taken in small doses for short periods of time. Never fall into the trap of thinking "if a little is good, more is better."

This section of the supplement charts also lists the available forms of the substance, even when a safe dosage cannot be recommended. Always follow the manufacturer's instructions and your doctor's advice.

N–Toxicity

This section includes a general, average toxicity rating for each medicinal herb and supplement.

O–Adverse Reactions, Side Effects or Overdose Symptoms

Adverse reactions or side effects are symptoms that may occur when you ingest any substance, whether it is food, medicine, mineral, supplement or vitamin. These are effects on the body other than the desired effect for which you take the substance.

The term *adverse reaction* means the reactions can cause hazards that outweigh benefits.

The term *side effect* may include an expected, perhaps unavoidable, effect of a mineral, supplement or vitamin. For example, a side effect of melatonin may be drowsiness the next morning. This symptom is harmless (unless extreme) and sometimes uncomfortable, but it has nothing to do with the intended use.

If you suspect an overdose, whether symptoms are present or not, follow the instructions in this section.

Checklist for Safer Use of Minerals, Supplements & Vitamins

The most important caution regarding all minerals, supplements and vitamins deals with the amount you take. Despite many popular articles in magazines and newspapers and reports on television, large doses of some of these substances can be hazardous to your health. Don't believe sensational advertisements and take large doses or megadoses. The belief "if a little does good, a lot will do much more" has no place in rational thinking regarding products to protect your health. Stay within safe-dose ranges!

1. Learn all you can about the minerals, supplements and vitamins *before* you take them. Information sources include this book, books from your public library, your doctor or your pharmacist.

2. Don't take minerals, supplements or vitamins prescribed for someone else, even if your symptoms are the same. At the same time, keep prescription items to yourself. They may be harmful to someone else.

3. Tell your doctor or health-care professional about any symptoms you experience that you suspect may be caused by anything you take.

4. Take minerals, supplements and vitamins in good light after you have identified the contents of the container. If you wear glasses, put them on to check and recheck labels.

5. Don't keep medicine by your bedside. You may unknowingly repeat a dose when you are half-asleep or confused.

6. Know the names of all the substances you take.

7. Read labels on medications you take. If the information is incomplete, ask your pharmacist for more details.

8. If the substance is in liquid form, shake it before you take it.

9. Store all minerals, supplements and vitamins in cool places away from sunlight and moisture. Bathroom medicine cabinets are usually unacceptable

because they are too warm and humid.

10. If a mineral, supplement or vitamin requires refrigeration, don't freeze!

11. Obtain a standard measuring spoon from your pharmacy for liquid substances and a graduated dropper to use for liquid preparations for infants and children.

12. Follow manufacturer's or doctor's suggestions regarding diet instructions. Some products work better on a full stomach. Others work best on an empty stomach. Some products work best when you follow a special diet. For example, a low-salt diet enhances effectiveness of any product expected to lower blood pressure.

13. Avoid any substance you know you are allergic to.

14. If you become pregnant while taking any mineral, supplement or vitamin, tell your physician and discontinue taking it until you have discussed it with him or her. Try to remember the exact dose and the length of time you have taken the substance.

15. Tell any healthcare provider about minerals, supplements, vitamins and other substances you take, even if you bought them without a prescription. During an illness or prior to surgery, this information is crucial. Even mention antacids, laxatives, tonics and over-the-counter preparations. Many people believe these products are completely safe and forget to inform doctors, nurses or pharmacists they are using them.

16. Regard all minerals, supplements and vitamins as potentially harmful to children. Store them safely away from their reach.

17. Alcohol, marijuana, cocaine, other mood-altering drugs and tobacco can cause life-threatening interactions when mixed with some minerals, supplements and vitamins. They can also prevent treatment from being effective or delay your return to good health. Common sense dictates you avoid them, particularly during an illness.

Minerals

Many minerals are essential parts of *enzymes*. They also actively participate in regulating many physiological functions: transporting oxygen to each of the body's cells, providing sparks to make muscles contract and participating in many ways to guarantee normal function of the central nervous system. Minerals are required for growth, maintenance, repair and health of tissues and bones.

Most minerals are widely distributed in foods. *Severe mineral deficiency is unusual in the United States and Canada.* As with vitamins, certain groups may be more likely to have a deficiency than others. For example: Pregnant women and children are at higher risk for iron deficiency, elderly persons are more at risk for zinc deficiency, and calcium requirements are increased for those at risk for osteoporosis.

Arsenic

 Basic Information

This metallic element is extremely poisonous.

- Available from natural sources? Yes
- Available from synthetic sources? No
- Prescription required? Yes, for some forms

 Natural Sources

Breads   Meats
Cereals   Starchy vegetables
Fish

 Benefits

- Arsenic is thought to be essential in trace amounts, but the benefits of this mineral are unknown.
- Arsenic is used in homeopathic treatment for some digestive problems that include burning pain and symptoms of dehydration.

 Possible Additional Benefits

Arsenic may help metabolize methionine.

 Who May Benefit from Additional Amounts?

Most individuals get an adequate amount from their diet.

 Deficiency Symptoms

No proven symptoms exist.

 Usage Information

What this mineral does:
- The exact function of arsenic is unclear, but it may aid methionine metabolism (methionine is an *amino acid*).
- Toxicity occurs in doses larger than 250mcg a day. Most diets contain about 140mcg a day.

Available as:
Arsenicum album (Ars alb), a dilute form of arsenic, is sometimes used to treat digestive problems. It is available as a liquid or tablet.

 Warnings and Precautions

Over 55:
Older persons may have a higher risk of excess arsenic due to decreased liver or kidney function.

Pregnancy: **Breastfeeding:**
Do not take.   Do not take.

Storage:
- Store safely out of reach of children.
- Store in a cool, dry place away from direct light, but don't freeze.
- Don't store in bathroom medicine cabinet. Heat and moisture may change the action of the mineral.

 Overdose/Toxicity

Signs and symptoms:
- Chronic symptoms include headaches, convulsion, confusion, drowsiness and change in fingernail color.

BORON 27

- Acute symptoms include vomiting, diarrhea, blood in urine, muscle cramps, fatigue, weakness, hair loss and dermatitis.
- Coma and death are possible when toxic arsenic levels accumulate.
- Lungs, skin, kidneys and liver are most affected by toxicity.
- Many types of cancer have been linked to arsenic exposure.

What to do:

For symptoms of overdose:
Discontinue mineral and consult doctor immediately. Also see *Adverse Reactions or Side Effects* section below.

For accidental overdose (such as child taking entire bottle): Dial 911 (emergency), 0 for operator or call your nearest Poison Control Center.

 Adverse Reactions or Side Effects

Reaction or effect	What to do
Blood in urine	Discontinue. Call doctor immediately.
Change in fingernail color	Discontinue. Call doctor immediately.
Confusion	Discontinue. Call doctor immediately.
Cramps	Discontinue. Call doctor immediately.
Dermatitis	Discontinue. Call doctor immediately.
Diarrhea	Discontinue. Call doctor immediately.
Drowsiness	Discontinue. Call doctor immediately.
Hair loss	Discontinue. Call doctor immediately.
Headaches	Discontinue. Call doctor immediately.
Nausea	Discontinue. Call doctor immediately.

 Interaction with Medicine, Minerals or Vitamins

Interacts with	Combined effect
Dimercaprol	Treats arsenic toxicity, especially in the first 24 hours after exposure.
Vitamin C	Defends (somewhat) against arsenic toxicity.

 Lab Tests to Detect Deficiency

Deficiency is determined by hair or blood tests.

Boron

 Basic Information

Boron is found in high concentrations in the parathyroid glands.

- Available from natural sources? Yes
- Available from synthetic sources? No
- Prescription required? No

 Natural Sources

Apples	Drinking Water	Leafy vegetables
Beer	(in certain areas)	Legumes
Carrots	Grains	Nuts
Cider	Grapes	Pears

 Benefits

- Important for preservation and development of bone
- Inhibits osteoporosis by halting demineralization (see Glossary) of bones
- Increases calcium absorption and metabolism
- Promotes normal growth and development

→

Possible
Additional Benefits

- May help treat osteoarthritis
- May improve immune system by boosting production of infection-fighting antibodies
- May treat arthritis pain and stiffness
- May reduce hypertension

 Who May Benefit
from Additional
Amounts?

Individuals at high risk for developing osteoporosis

 Deficiency
Symptoms

Poor bone development

 Usage Information

What this mineral does:

- Necessary element for plants
- Important for mineral and energy metabolism
- Regulates hormones
- Important for bone growth and maintenance
- Contributes to health of cell membranes
- Aids some enzyme reactions

Miscellaneous information:

Boric acid is commonly used as an eye wash and antiseptic for the skin.

Available as:

- Individual supplement
- A constituent of some multivitamins

 Warnings and
Precautions

Consult your doctor if you have:

- Osteoporosis
- Hypercalcemia

Pregnancy:
Consult your doctor.

Breastfeeding:
Consult your doctor.

Storage:

- Store safely out of reach of children.
- Store in a cool, dry place away from direct light, but don't freeze.
- Don't store in bathroom medicine cabinet. Heat and moisture may change the action of the mineral.

 Overdose/Toxicity

Signs and symptoms:

Nausea, vomiting, hair loss, skin rash, lethargy, headache, diarrhea, hypothermia, restlessness, kidney damage, circulatory collapse and shock leading to death

What to do:

For symptoms of overdose:
Discontinue mineral and consult doctor immediately. Also see *Adverse Reactions or Side Effects* section below.

For accidental overdose (such as child taking entire bottle): Dial 911 (emergency), 0 for operator or call your nearest Poison Control Center.

 Adverse Reactions
or Side Effects

Reaction or effect	What to do
Appetite loss	Discontinue. Call doctor when convenient.
Nausea	Discontinue. Call doctor when convenient.
Weight loss	Discontinue. Call doctor when convenient.

Interaction with Medicine, Minerals or Vitamins

Interacts with	Combined effect
Calcium	Aids metabolism of calcium.
Magnesium	Aids metabolism of magnesium.
Phosphorus	Aids metabolism of phosphorus.

 Lab Tests to Detect Deficiency

None are available.

Calcium

 Basic Information

Calcium citrate and *calcium gluconate* are common forms of calcium supplements.

- Available from natural sources? Yes
- Available from synthetic sources? Yes
- Prescription required? Yes, for some forms
- *Optimal Intake,* see pages 182–183

 Natural Sources

Almonds	Kelp
Brazil nuts	Milk
Broccoli	Pudding
Calcium-fortified cereal, rice, juice	Salmon, canned
	Sardines, canned
Caviar	Turnip greens
Cheese	Yogurt
Cottage cheese	

 Benefits

- Helps prevent osteoporosis
- Treats calcium depletion in people with hypoparathyroidism, osteomalacia, rickets
- Used medically to treat tetany (severe muscle spasms) caused by sensitivity reactions, cardiac arrest, lead poisoning
- Used medically as an antidote to magnesium poisoning
- Prevents muscle or leg cramps in some people
- Promotes normal growth and development
- Builds bones and teeth
- Maintains bone density and strength
- Buffers acid in stomach and acts as antacid
- Helps regulate heartbeat, blood clotting, muscle contraction
- Treats neonatal hypocalcemia
- Promotes storage and release of some body hormones
- Lowers phosphate concentrations in people with chronic kidney disease
- Helps reduce blood pressure in certain people

 Possible Additional Benefits

- May help decrease risk of kidney stones
- Potential treatment for toxemia in pregnant women
- May reduce the risk of colon cancer

→

Who May Benefit from Additional Amounts?

- Anyone with inadequate caloric or dietary intake or increased nutritional requirements or those who do not like or consume milk products
- People allergic to milk and milk products
- People with untreated lactase deficiency who avoid milk and dairy products
- People over 55 years old, particularly women
- Women throughout adult life, especially during pregnancy and lactation, but not limited to these times
- Those who abuse alcohol or other drugs
- People with a chronic wasting illness
- Those under excess stress for long periods
- Anyone who has recently undergone surgery
- People with bone fractures
- Adolescents with low dietary calcium intake

Deficiency Symptoms

Osteoporosis (late symptoms):
- Frequent fractures in spine and other bones
- Deformed spinal column with humps
- Loss of height

Osteomalacia:
- Frequent fractures
- Muscle contractions
- Convulsive seizures
- Muscle cramps

Usage Information

What this mineral does:
- Participates in metabolic functions necessary for normal activity of nervous, muscular, skeletal systems
- Plays important role in normal heart function, kidney function, blood clotting, blood-vessel integrity
- Helps utilize vitamin B-12

Miscellaneous information:
- Bones serve as a storage site for calcium in the body. There is a constant interchange between calcium in bone and in the bloodstream.
- Foods rich in calcium (or supplements) help maintain the balance between bone needs and blood needs.
- Exercise, a balanced diet, calcium from natural sources or supplements and estrogens are important in treating and preventing osteoporosis.
- The aluminum found in some antacids may interfere with the absorption of calcium.
- Recent studies indicate that bone mineral content is increased when calcium supplements are given during adolescence.
- Those who live in geographic areas with low sun exposure and home-bound or institutionalized persons should take vitamin D with calcium to improve absorption.

Available as:
- Tablets: Swallow whole with a full glass of liquid. Don't chew or crush. Take with or 1 to 1-1/2 hours after meals unless otherwise directed by your doctor.
- Chewable tablets: Chew well before swallowing.
- Calcium is available as carbonate, citrate and gluconate, with varying levels of bioavailability (see Glossary).

Warnings and Precautions

Don't take if you:

- Are allergic to calcium or antacids
- Have a high blood-calcium level
- Have sarcoidosis

Consult your doctor if you have:

- Kidney disease
- Chronic constipation, colitis, diarrhea
- Stomach or intestinal bleeding
- Irregular heartbeat
- Heart problems or high blood pressure for which you are taking a calcium channel blocker

Over 55:

- Adverse reactions and side effects are more likely.
- Diarrhea or constipation are particularly likely.

Pregnancy:

- Pregnant women may need extra calcium. Consult your doctor about supplements.
- Don't take megadoses (see *Optimal Daily Intake Information*, page 182).

Breastfeeding:

- The drug passes into milk. Consult your doctor about supplements.
- Don't take megadoses (see *Optimal Daily Intake Information*, page 182).

Effect on lab tests:

- Serum-amylase and serum-11 hydroxycorticosteroid concentrations can be increased.
- Excessive, prolonged use decreases serum-phosphate concentration.

Storage:

- Store in cool, dry place away from direct light, but don't freeze.
- Store safely out of reach of children.
- Don't store in bathroom medicine cabinet. Heat and moisture may change the action of the mineral.

Others:

- Dolomite and bone meal are probably unsafe sources of calcium because they contain lead.
- Avoid taking calcium within 1 or 2 hours of meals or ingestion of other medicines, if possible.
- Some calcium carbonate is derived from oyster shells. Calcium carbonate derived from this source is not recommended!

Overdose/Toxicity

Signs and symptoms:

- Confusion, slow or irregular heartbeat, bone or muscle pain, nausea, vomiting
- Signs and symptoms of toxicity have not been seen, even at doses of 2 to 3 grams/day

What to do:

For symptoms of overdose: Discontinue mineral and consult doctor immediately. Also see *Adverse Reactions or Side Effects* section below.

For accidental overdose (such as child taking entire bottle): Dial 911 (emergency), 0 for operator or call your nearest Poison Control Center.

Adverse Reactions or Side Effects

Reaction or effect	What to do
Early signs of too much calcium in blood:	
Constipation	Increase fluid intake. Discontinue. Call doctor when convenient.
Headache	Discontinue. Call doctor when convenient.
Late signs of too much calcium in blood:	
Confusion	Discontinue. Call doctor immediately.

MINERALS

→

Muscle or bone pain	Discontinue. Call doctor immediately.
Nausea or vomiting	Discontinue. Call doctor immediately.
Slow or irregular heartbeat	Seek emergency treatment.

Interaction with Medicine, Minerals or Vitamins

Interacts with	Combined effect
Cellulose sodium phosphate	Decreases effect of cellulose sodium phosphate.
Digitalis preparations	Causes heartbeat irregularities.
Etidronate	Decreases effects of etidronate. Don't take within 2 hours of calcium supplements.
Gallium nitrate	Inhibits function of gallium nitrate.
Iron supplements	Decreases absorption of iron unless vitamin C is taken at the same time.
Magnesium-containing medications or supplements	Increases absorption of magnesium and calcium.
Oral contraceptives and estrogens	May increase calcium absorption.
Phenytoin	Decreases effect of both calcium and phenytoin. Do not take calcium within 1 to 3 hours of phenytoin.
Tetracyclines (oral)	Decreases absorption of tetracycline.
Vitamin D	Increases absorption of calcium supplements.

Interaction with Other Substances

Alcohol decreases absorption.

Beverages:
Caffeine (coffee, tea, cola, chocolate) can decrease absorption but has not been shown to decrease bone density.

Lab Tests to Detect Deficiency

- 24-hour urine collection to measure calcium levels (Sulkowitch)
- Imaging procedures to scan for bone density (more reliable than above test)

Chloride

Basic Information
• Available from natural sources? Yes
• Available from synthetic sources? Yes
• Prescription required? No

Natural Sources
Salt substitutes (potassium chloride)
Sea salt
Table salt (sodium chloride)
Note: Chloride is found in combination with other molecules.

Benefits
• Regulates body's electrolyte (see Glossary) balance
• Regulates body's acid-base balance
• Promotes nerve and muscle function

Possible Additional Benefits
None are known.

Who May Benefit from Additional Amounts?
• People with Bartter's syndrome
• Individuals with renal tubular disorders or cystic fibrosis

Deficiency Symptoms
Note: Chloride deficiency is basically unheard of in the United States except in people with acute acid-base disorders.

Causes:
• Continuous vomiting can lead to a deficiency.
• When chloride is intentionally neglected in infant-formula preparations, the infant develops metabolic alkalosis, hypovolemia and significant urinary loss. Psychomotor defects, memory loss and growth retardation also occur. This is not a problem with commercially available formulas.

Symptoms:
• Upset balance of acids and bases in body fluids (rare)
• Nausea
• Vomiting
• Confusion
• Weakness
• Coma

Usage Information
What this mineral does:
• Chloride is a constituent of acid in the stomach (hydrochloric acid).
• It interacts with sodium, potassium and carbon dioxide to maintain acid-base balance in body cells and fluids. It is crucial to normal health.
• Concentrations of sodium, potassium, carbon dioxide and chlorine are controlled by mechanisms inside each body cell.

Miscellaneous information:
• Healthy people do not have to make any special efforts to maintain sufficient chloride.
• Eating a balanced diet supplies all daily needs.

MINERALS

→

- Extremely ill patients, with acid-base imbalance, require hospitalization, frequent lab studies and skillful professional care.

Available as:

- Sodium-chloride (salt) tablets: These may cause stomach distress and overload on kidneys.
- Chloride is a constituent of many multivitamin/mineral preparations.

 Warnings and Precautions

Chloride supplement is not warranted except with significant alterations in acid-base balance, which would require medical care.

 Overdose/Toxicity

Signs and symptoms:

- Upset in balance of acids and bases in body fluids can occur with too much chloride or with too little chloride. Symptoms of either include weakness, confusion and coma.
- Consumption of reasonable amounts of chloride in the form of table salt or potassium replacement is not problematic.

What to do:

For symptoms of overdose: Discontinue mineral and consult doctor.

For accidental overdose (such as child taking a large amount): Dial 911 (emergency), 0 for operator or call your nearest Poison Control Center.

 Adverse Reactions or Side Effects

None are expected.

 Interaction with Medicine, Minerals or Vitamins

Interacts with	Combined effect
Chlorine	Maintains normal acid-base balance in body.
Potassium	Maintains normal acid-base balance in body.
Sodium	Maintains normal acid-base balance in body.

 Lab Tests to Detect Deficiency

Serum chloride

Chromium

Basic Information
- Available from natural sources? Yes
- Available from synthetic sources? No
- Prescription required? No
- *Optimal Intake,* see pages 182–183

Natural Sources

Apples	Eggs
Beef	Ham
Brewer's yeast	Molasses
Broccoli	Sweet potatoes
Calf liver	Tomatoes
Cheese	Whole-grain
Chicken	products
Corn on the cob	

Benefits
- Decreases total cholesterol and LDL (see Glossary)
- Promotes glucose metabolism
- Helps insulin regulate blood sugar
- Decreases insulin requirements and improves glucose tolerance of some people with type II diabetes
- Aids protein synthesis

Possible Additional Benefits
Possible weight loss and increase in muscle tissue

Who May Benefit from Additional Amounts?
- Those who abuse alcohol or other drugs
- People with a chronic wasting illness
- Anyone who has recently undergone surgery
- Possibly diabetics

Deficiency Symptoms
- Reduced tissue sensitivity to glucose, similar to diabetes
- Disturbances of glucose, fat and protein metabolism
- Numbness in extremities

Usage Information

What this mineral does:
- Aids transport of glucose into cells
- Enhances effect of insulin in glucose utilization

Miscellaneous information:
- Chromium toxicity can result from industrial overexposure, such as tanning, electroplating, steel making, abrasives manufacturing, cement manufacturing, diesel-locomotive repairs, furniture polishing, fur processing, glass making, jewelry making, metal cleaning, oil drilling, photography, textile dyeing and wood preservative manufacturing.
- Nutritional science has yet to determine the exact amounts of chromium in most foods. Less than 1% of dietary chromium is absorbed.

Available as:
- A constituent of many multivitamin/mineral preparations
- An individualized supplement

MINERALS

→

Warnings and Precautions

Don't take if you:
Work in an environment that has high concentrations of chromium.

Consult your doctor if you have:
• Diabetes
• Lung disease
• Liver disease
• Kidney disease

Over 55:
No special needs if you eat a balanced diet.

Pregnancy:
Avoid chromium during pregnancy until further information is available.

Breastfeeding:
Avoid chromium during breastfeeding until further information is available.

Effect on lab tests:
Diagnostic tests, such as red-blood-cell-survival studies performed after radioactive-hexavalent chromium is used for 3 months, may cause falsely elevated levels in blood.

Storage:
• Store in cool, dry place away from direct light, but don't freeze.
• Store safely out of reach of children.
• Don't store in bathroom medicine cabinet. Heat and moisture may change the action of the mineral.

 ## Overdose/Toxicity

Signs and symptoms:
The dietary form has very low toxicity. Long-term exposure to environmental chromium may lead to skin problems, liver impairment or kidney impairment.

What to do:
For symptoms of overdose:
Discontinue mineral and consult doctor.

For accidental overdose (such as child taking entire bottle): Dial 911 (emergency), 0 for operator or call your nearest Poison Control Center.

 ## Adverse Reactions or Side Effects

None are expected.

 ## Interaction with Medicine, Minerals or Vitamins

Interacts with	Combined effect
Insulin	May decrease amount of insulin needed to treat diabetes if taken at high levels.

 ## Lab Tests to Detect Deficiency

• Serum chromium
• Hair analysis not reliable test for deficiency or toxicity

Cobalt

Basic Information

- Available from natural sources? Yes
- Available from synthetic sources? Yes
- Prescription required? No, but supplements are hard to find, so adequate food intake is important.

Natural Sources

Clams	Liver
Dairy products	Meats
Kidney	Oysters

Note: Small amounts in diet satisfy requirements, except under unusual circumstances. Small amounts exist in some plant foods but are best utilized as part of B-12-rich foods.

Benefits

- Promotes normal red-blood-cell formation
- Constituent of B-12
- Involved in enzyme reactions
- Aids in forming myelin nerve coverings

Possible Additional Benefits

- May play a role in treating anemia that does not respond to other treatment
- May treat fatigue, digestive disorders and neuromuscular problems
- May treat certain cancers (radioactive cobalt-60)

Who May Benefit from Additional Amounts?

- People with recent severe burns or injuries
- Those with anorexia nervosa or bulimia
- Vegan vegetarians with inadequate B-12 intake

Deficiency Symptoms

Pernicious anemia, with the following symptoms:

- Weakness, especially in arms and legs
- Sore tongue
- Nausea, appetite loss, weight loss
- Bleeding gums
- Numbness and tingling in hands and feet
- Difficulty maintaining balance
- Pale lips, tongue, gums
- Confusion and dementia
- Headache
- Poor memory

Usage Information

What this mineral does:

Cobalt acts as a catalyst in complex reactions to form vitamin B-12.

Miscellaneous information:

- Cobalt is a trace element stored mainly in the liver.
- Deficiency is extremely rare.
- It is a necessary ingredient to manufacture vitamin B-12 in the body. A deficiency of cobalt may lead to a deficiency of vitamin B-12 and therefore to pernicious anemia.

Available as:

Capsules: Swallow whole with a full glass of liquid. Don't chew or crush. Take with or 1 to 1-1/2 hours after meals unless otherwise directed by your doctor.

MINERALS

Warnings and Precautions

Over 55:
Eat a balanced diet to prevent deficiency.

Pregnancy:
Take as B-12 if your doctor advises.

Breastfeeding:
Take as B-12 if your doctor advises.

Storage:
- Store in cool, dry place away from direct light, but don't freeze.
- Store safely out of reach of children.
- Don't store in bathroom medicine cabinet. Heat and moisture may change the action of the mineral.

 Overdose/Toxicity

Signs and symptoms:
- In large doses (20–30mg/day), cobalt can produce polycythemia, enlargement of thyroid gland and enlargement of the heart leading to congestive heart failure (see Glossary).
- Cobalt toxicity can cause thyroid overgrowth in infants.

What to do:
For symptoms of overdose:
Discontinue mineral and consult doctor. Also see *Adverse Reactions or Side Effects* section below.

For accidental overdose (such as child taking large amounts): Dial 911 (emergency), 0 for operator or call your nearest Poison Control Center.

 Adverse Reactions or Side Effects

Reaction or effect	What to do
With megadoses:	
Enlargement of heart	Discontinue. Call doctor immediately.
Enlargement of thyroid gland	Discontinue. Call doctor immediately.
Polycythemia	Discontinue. Call doctor immediately.

 Interaction with Medicine, Minerals or Vitamins

Interacts with	Combined effect
Colchicine	May cause inaccurate lab studies of cobalt or vitamin B-12.
Neomycin	May cause inaccurate lab studies of cobalt or vitamin B-12.
Para-aminosalicylic acid	May cause inaccurate lab studies of cobalt or vitamin B-12.
Phenytoin	May cause inaccurate lab studies of cobalt or vitamin B-12.

 Interaction with Other Substances

Some beer contains cobalt as a stabilizer. People who consume large quantities of cobalt-stabilized beer over long periods may develop cobalt toxicity leading to cardiomyopathy (see Glossary) and congestive heart failure (see Glossary).

 Lab Tests to Detect Deficiency

- Concentration in human plasma
- Measured in bioassay as part of vitamin B-12

Copper

Basic Information

- Available from natural sources? Yes
- Available from synthetic sources? No
- Prescription required? No
- *Optimal Intake,* see pages 182–183

Natural Sources

Avocados   Oats
Fish   Oysters
Legumes   Peanuts
Lentils   Raisins
Liver   Salmon
Lobster   Shellfish
Mushrooms   Soybeans
Nuts   Spinach

Note: Copper-bottom pans and pipes can also raise the copper content of water and food supply.

Benefits

- Promotes normal red-blood-cell formation
- Acts as a catalyst in storage and release of iron to form hemoglobin for red blood cells
- Assists in production of several enzymes involved in respiration
- Promotes connective-tissue formation and central-nervous-system function
- Assists in production of several enzymes involved in forming melanin
- Promotes normal insulin function
- Helps maintain myelin
- Part of superoxide dismutase and its antioxidant (see Glossary) capacity

Possible Additional Benefits

- May be used to treat nutritional anemias along with iron, B-12 and/or folate
- May protect against cardiovascular disease; however, balance is critical because high levels of copper have been seen in patients with cardiovascular disease
- Possibly reduces inflammation associated with arthritis
- May enhance immune function

Who May Benefit from Additional Amounts?

- Anyone with inadequate caloric or dietary intake or increased nutritional requirements
- People over 55 years old
- Those who abuse alcohol or other drugs
- People with a chronic wasting illness, particularly those with chronic diarrhea, malabsorption disorders (see Glossary), kidney disease
- Anyone on long-term zinc supplementation
- People with recent severe burns or injuries

Deficiency Symptoms

- Anemia
- Low white-blood-cell count associated with reduced resistance to infection
- Faulty collagen formation
- Bone demineralization (see Glossary)
- Loss of hair, skin pigmentation

MINERALS

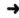

Usage Information

What this mineral does:
Copper is an essential component of a number of proteins and enzymes, including lysyl, hydroxylase and dopamine beta-hydroxylase.

Miscellaneous information:
- Plasma-copper levels may increase in people with rheumatoid arthritis, pregnancy, cirrhosis of the liver, myocardial infarction (heart attack), schizophrenia, tumors or severe infections.
- Copper supplementation of 2mg/day is recommended for people on long-term zinc therapy supplementation.
- Menkes syndrome is a genetic defect in copper metabolism, which requires medical intervention.
- Processed foods may reduce normal copper absorption.
- Plasma-copper levels decrease with hypothyroidism, neutropenia, leukopenia, kwashiorkor, sprue and nephrosis.
- Most nutritionists recommend a balanced diet rather than extra supplementation that could upset the body's delicate mineral balance.

Available as:
- Tablets: Swallow whole with a full glass of liquid. Don't chew or crush. Take with or 1 to 1-1/2 hours after meals unless otherwise directed by your doctor.
- Copper is a constituent of many multivitamin/mineral preparations.

Warnings and Precautions

Don't take if you:
Have Wilson's disease.

Consult your doctor if you are:
Considering taking a copper supplement.

Pregnancy:
Consult your doctor.

Breastfeeding:
Consult your doctor.

Effect on lab tests:
Cobalt, iron, nickel and oral contraceptives with estrogens can cause false-positive or elevated copper values.

Storage:
- Store in cool, dry place away from direct light, but don't freeze.
- Store safely out of reach of children.
- Don't store in bathroom medicine cabinet. Heat and moisture may change the action of the mineral.

Overdose/Toxicity

Signs and symptoms:
Nausea, vomiting, muscle aches, abdominal pain, anemia

What to do:
For symptoms of overdose:
Discontinue mineral and consult doctor.

For accidental overdose (such as child taking entire bottle): Dial 911 (emergency), 0 for operator or call your nearest Poison Control Center.

Adverse Reactions or Side Effects

None are expected.

Interaction with Medicine, Minerals or Vitamins

Interacts with	Combined effect
Cadmium	May interfere with copper absorption and utilization.
Fiber	May interfere with copper absorption and utilization. Not clinically significant.
Molybdenum	Maintains appropriate ratio of copper to molybdenum in body. If you have excessive amounts of copper, your molybdenum level drops. If you have excessive amounts of molybdenum, your copper level drops.
Oral contraceptives	Increases copper level. Significance unknown at present.
Phytates (cereals, vegetables)	May interfere with copper absorption and utilization. Not clinically significant.
Vitamin C	Decreases absorption of copper. Large doses of vitamin C must be taken to produce this effect.
Zinc	May interfere with copper absorption and utilization. Copper supplement advised.

Lab Tests to Detect Deficiency

- Plasma-copper levels
- Urine-copper levels in 24-hour collection

MINERALS

Fluoride

Basic Information

Fluoride is available commercially as *sodium fluoride.*

- Available from natural sources? Yes
- Available from synthetic sources? Yes
- Prescription required? Yes, for some forms
- *Optimal Intake,* see pages 182–183

Natural Sources

Apples	Salmon, canned
Calf liver	Sardines, canned
Cod	Tea
Eggs	Water (does not
Kidney	include bottled water)

Note: The fluoride content of foods varies tremendously. It is relatively high where soils are rich and water is fluoridated and low otherwise.

Benefits

- Prevents dental caries (cavities) in children when level of fluoride in water is inadequate
- Treats osteoporosis with calcium and vitamin D, but use must be carefully monitored by a physician

Possible Additional Benefits

May play a role in preventing osteoporosis

→

Who May Benefit from Additional Amounts?

People living in an area with low-fluoride water content (check with your doctor, dentist or local health department)

Deficiency Symptoms

Significant increase in dental cavities

Usage Information

What this mineral does:

- Contributes to solid bone and tooth formation by helping body retain calcium
- Interferes with growth and development of bacteria that cause dental plaque

Miscellaneous information:

- Taking fluoride does not remove the need for good dental habits, including a good diet, brushing and flossing teeth and regular dental visits.
- If fluoride supplementation is needed in your area, continue until your child is 16. Subsequent topical applications every year or two may be continued to prevent cavities.

Available as:

- Tablets: Swallow whole with a full glass of liquid. Don't chew or crush. Take with or 1 to 1-1/2 hours after meals unless otherwise directed by your doctor.
- Drops: Dilute in at least 1/2 glass of water or other liquid. Take with or 1 to 1-1/2 hours after meals unless otherwise directed by your doctor. Do not take with milk or dairy products.

- Rinses: Follow directions and use just before bedtime, after proper brushing and flossing.
- Gels: Follow directions and use just before bedtime, after proper brushing and flossing.
- Paste: Follow directions and use just before bedtime, after proper brushing and flossing.

Warnings and Precautions

Don't take if:

Fluoride intake from drinking water exceeds 0.7 parts fluoride/million. Too much fluoride stains teeth permanently (fluorosis).

Consult your doctor if you have:

- Osteoporosis
- Underactive thyroid function

Pregnancy:

Reports do not agree on benefit and risk to unborn child. Follow your doctor's instructions.

Breastfeeding:

Consult your doctor. Infant supplementation may be advised.

Effect on lab tests:

- Serum acid phosphatase, serum calcium and protein-bound iodine may be falsely decreased.
- Serum aspartate aminotransferase—SGOT (see Glossary)—may be falsely increased.

Storage:

- Store in cool, dry place away from direct light, but don't freeze.
- Keep in original plastic container. Fluoride decomposes glass.
- Store safely out of reach of children.
- Don't store in bathroom medicine cabinet. Heat and moisture may change the action of the mineral.

Overdose/Toxicity

Signs and symptoms:

- Stomach cramps or pain, faintness, vomiting (possibly bloody), diarrhea, black stools, shallow breathing, tremors, increased saliva, unusual excitement
- Whitish streaks or patches or brown streaking (dental fluorosis) in children whose tooth enamel is not completely formed

What to do:

For symptoms of overdose:
Discontinue mineral and consult doctor. Also see *Adverse Reactions or Side Effects* section below.

For accidental overdose (such as child taking entire bottle): Dial 911 (emergency), 0 for operator or call your nearest Poison Control Center.

Adverse Reactions or Side Effects

Reaction or effect	What to do
With excessive amounts of fluoride:	
Appetite loss	Discontinue. Call doctor when convenient.
Constipation	Discontinue. Call doctor when convenient.
Mottling of teeth with brown, black or white discoloration	Discontinue. Call doctor when convenient.
Nausea	Discontinue. Call doctor when convenient.
Skin rash	Discontinue. Call doctor immediately.

Interaction with Medicine, Minerals or Vitamins

Interacts with	Combined effect
Aluminum hydroxide	Decreases absorption of fluoride.
Calcium supplements	Decreases absorption of fluoride.

Interaction with Other Substances

Beverages: Milk decreases absorption of fluoride. Take dose 2 hours before or after drinking milk.

Lab Tests to Detect Deficiency

None are available. Examinations of mouth for dental cavities once or twice a year yield all necessary evidence.

MINERALS

Germanium

Basic Information

The oil form is used in aromatherapy.

- Available from natural sources? Yes
- Available from synthetic sources? Yes
- Prescription required? No

Natural Sources

Aloe vera	Ginseng
Comfrey	Onions
Chlorella	Shiitake mushrooms
Garlic	Suma

Benefits

Boosts oxygenation (see Glossary) of tissue

Possible Additional Benefits

- May aid immune system
- May help rid the body of toxins and poisons
- Possible treatment for rheumatoid arthritis
- May treat food allergies
- Potential treatment for candidiasis
- May promote wound healing
- Oil form may be useful in treating wounds and burns, stress, menopausal and menstrual difficulties, athlete's foot, eczema, shingles, sore throat, mouth ulcers, insect stings, headaches, hemorrhoids

Who May Benefit from Additional Amounts?

Those with immune suppression

Deficiency Symptoms

No proven symptoms exist.

Usage Information

What this mineral does:

Germanium is involved in cellular oxygenation (see Glossary).

Miscellaneous information:

- Used to make computer chips
- Best taken by eating foods rich in germanium

Available as:

- Tablets: Take as directed by manufacturer or your doctor.
- Powder: Take as directed by manufacturer or your doctor.
- Capsules: Take as directed by manufacturer or your doctor.
- Oil: Take as directed by manufacturer or your doctor.
- "Organic" form: 25 mg/day (GE-132)—other forms may cause kidney damage.

Warnings and Precautions

Pregnancy: **Breastfeeding:**
Do not use.   Do not use.

Storage:

- Store in a cool, dry place away from direct light, but don't freeze.
- Store safely out of reach of children.
- Don't store in bathroom medicine cabinet. Heat and moisture may change the action of the mineral.

Others:
Do not use oils around eyes.

Overdose/Toxicity

Signs and symptoms:
Large doses may harm kidneys, liver, muscles, nerves and brain.

What to do:
For symptoms of overdose:
Discontinue mineral and consult doctor immediately.

For accidental overdose (such as child taking entire bottle): Dial 911 (emergency), 0 for operator or call your nearest Poison Control Center.

Adverse Reactions or Side Effects

None are expected.

Interaction with Medicine, Minerals or Vitamins

None are known.

Lab Tests to Detect Deficiency

None are available.

MINERALS

Iodine

Basic Information

• Available from natural sources? Yes
• Available from synthetic sources? No
• Prescription required? Yes, for strengths over 130mg
• *Optimal Intake*, see pages 182-183

Natural Sources

Lobster	Saltwater fish
Milk	(cod, haddock,
Nutritional yeast	herring)
Oysters	Sea salt
Salmon, canned	Seaweed
Salted nuts, seeds,	Shrimp
snack foods	Table salt (iodized)

Benefits

• Promotes normal function of thyroid gland
• Promotes normal cell function
• Shrinks thyroid prior to thyroid surgery
• Tests thyroid function before and after administration of a radioactive form of iodine
• Keeps skin, hair, nails healthy
• Prevents goiter

Possible Additional Benefits

None are known.

→

Who May Benefit from Additional Amounts?

Anyone who lives in a region where the soil is deficient in iodine (deficiency is usually treated by using iodized table salt)

Deficiency Symptoms

Children:
• Depressed growth
• Delayed sexual development
• Mental retardation
• Deafness

Adults:
Goiter

Symptoms of low thyroid-hormone level (children and adults):
• Listlessness
• Sluggish behavior

Usage Information

What this mineral does:
Iodine is an integral part of the thyroid hormones tetraiodothyronine (thyroxin) and triiodothyronine.

Miscellaneous information:
Iodized salt and the use of iodophors as antiseptics by the dairy industry are the main source of iodine in most diets.

Available as:
• Tablets: Swallow whole with a full glass of liquid. Don't chew or crush. Take with or 1 to 1-1/2 hours after meals unless otherwise directed by your doctor.
• Oral solution: Dilute in at least 1/2 glass of water or other liquid.

Take with or 1 to 1-1/2 hours after meals unless otherwise directed by your doctor.
• Enteric-coated tablets are not recommended. They may cause obstruction, bleeding and perforation of the small bowel.

Warnings and Precautions

Don't take if you have:
• Elevated serum potassium (determined by lab study)
• Myotonia congenita

Consult your doctor if you have:
• Hyperthyroidism
• Kidney disease
• Taken or are taking amiloride, antithyroid medications, lithium, spironolactone, triamterene

Pregnancy:
If you consume too much iodine during pregnancy, the infant may have thyroid enlargement, hypothyroidism or cretinism (dwarfism and mental deficiency).

Breastfeeding:
• Avoid supplements while nursing.
• Iodine in milk can cause skin rash and suppression of normal thyroid function in infant.

Effect on lab tests:
• May cause false elevation in all thyroid-function studies
• Interferes with test for naturally occurring steroids in urine

Storage:
• Store in cool, dry place away from direct light, but don't freeze.
• Store safely out of reach of children.
• Don't store in bathroom medicine cabinet. Heat and moisture may change the action of the mineral.

Overdose/Toxicity

Signs and symptoms:
Irregular heartbeat; confusion; difficulty breathing; swollen neck or throat; bloody or black, tarry stools

What to do:
For symptoms of overdose:
Discontinue mineral and consult doctor. Also see *Adverse Reactions or Side Effects* section below.

For accidental overdose (such as child taking entire bottle): Dial 911 (emergency), 0 for operator or call your nearest Poison Control Center.

 Adverse Reactions or Side Effects

Reaction or effect   What to do

Note: These reactions are all rare.

Reaction or effect	What to do
Abdominal pain	Discontinue. Call doctor immediately.
Burning in mouth or throat	Discontinue. Call doctor immediately.
Diarrhea	Discontinue. Call doctor immediately.
Fever	Discontinue. Call doctor immediately.
Headache	Discontinue. Call doctor immediately.
Heavy legs	Discontinue. Call doctor when convenient.
Increased salivation	Discontinue. Call doctor immediately.
Metallic taste	Discontinue. Call doctor when convenient.
Nausea	Continue. Tell doctor at next visit.
Numbness, tingling or pain in hands or feet	Discontinue. Call doctor immediately.
Skin rash	Discontinue. Call doctor immediately.
Sore teeth or gums	Discontinue. Call doctor immediately.
Swelling of salivary gland	Seek emergency treatment.
Tiredness or weakness	Discontinue. Call doctor immediately.

 Interaction with Medicine, Minerals or Vitamins

Interacts with	Combined effect
Lithium carbonate for manic-depressive illness	Produces abnormally low thyroid activity. People taking lithium carbonate should avoid iodine, which suppresses the thyroid gland.

 Lab Tests to Detect Deficiency

Tests may indicate lower than normal thyroid function, implying a deficiency of iodine in some cases.

MINERALS

Iron

Basic Information

Ferrous sulfate is the most common form of iron.

- Available from natural sources? Yes
- Available from synthetic sources? Yes
- Prescription required? Yes, for some forms
- *Optimal Intake,* see pages 182–183

Natural Sources

Bread, enriched	Mussels
Egg yolk	Oysters
Fish	Red meats
Garbanzo beans	Seaweed, greens
(chickpeas)	Whole-grain
Lentils	products, enriched
Liver	

Molasses, blackstrap

Note: Only about 10% of food iron is absorbed from food consumed by an individual with normal iron stores; however, an iron-deficient person may absorb 20% to 30%.

Benefits

- Prevents and treats iron-deficiency anemia due to dietary iron deficiency or other causes
- Stimulates bone-marrow production of hemoglobin, the red-blood-cell pigment that carries oxygen to body cells
- Forms part of several enzymes and proteins in the body

Possible Additional Benefits

- May help alleviate menstrual discomfort
- May stimulate immunity in iron-deficient people
- May promote learning in children with iron deficiency

Who May Benefit from Additional Amounts?

- Many women, of child-bearing age, with heavy menstrual flow and women with long menstrual periods or short menstrual cycles (common in teenage girls)
- Anyone with inadequate caloric or dietary intake or increased nutritional requirements
- People over 55 years old
- Pregnant or breastfeeding women
- Those who abuse alcohol or other drugs
- People with a chronic wasting illness
- Those under excess stress for long periods
- Anyone who has recently undergone surgery
- Athletes and workers who participate in vigorous physical activities
- Anyone who has lost blood recently, such as from heavy menstrual periods, an accident or long-term, undetected gastrointestinal bleeding
- Vegetarians with inadequate dietary intake
- Infants from 2 to 24 months

Deficiency Symptoms

- Listlessness
- Heart palpitations upon exertion
- Fatigue
- Irritability
- Pale appearance to skin, mucous membranes, nails
- Decreased mental capacity, learning deficit
- Pica

Usage Information

What this mineral does:

- Iron is an essential component of hemoglobin, myoglobin and a cofactor (see Glossary) of several essential enzymes. Of the total iron in the body, 60% to 70% is stored in hemoglobin (the red part of red blood cells).
- Hemoglobin is also a component of myoglobin, an iron-protein complex in muscles. This complex helps muscles get extra energy when they work hard.

Miscellaneous information:

- Iron-deficiency anemia in older men is usually due to a slow loss of blood.
- Iron content of foods, especially acidic foods, can be dramatically increased when prepared in iron cookware.
- You may require 3 weeks of treatment before you receive the maximum benefit.
- Vitamin C (ascorbic acid) enhances iron absorption.
- Elevated iron levels have been associated with a high risk of heart disease.

Available as:

- Tablets and capsules: Swallow whole with a full glass of liquid. Don't chew

or crush. Take with food or immediately after eating to decrease stomach irritation.
- Oral solution: Dilute in at least 1/2 glass of water or other liquid. Take with or 1 to 1-1/2 hours after meals unless otherwise directed by your doctor.
- Chewable tablets: Chew well before swallowing.
- Enteric-coated tablets: Swallow whole with a full glass of liquid. Take with meals or 1 to 1-1/2 hours after meals unless otherwise directed by your doctor.

Warnings and Precautions

Don't take if you have:

- An allergy to any iron supplement
- Acute hepatitis
- Hemosiderosis or hemochromatosis (conditions involving excess iron in body)
- Hemolytic anemia
- Had repeated blood transfusions

Consult your doctor if you have:

- Plans to become pregnant while taking medication
- Had peptic-ulcer disease, enteritis, colitis
- Had pancreatitis or hepatitis
- Had a history of coronary artery disease
- Alcoholism
- Kidney disease
- Intestinal disease
- Excess vitamin C—problematic in people with iron-storage disorder

Over 55:

- Deficiency is not uncommon. Check frequently with your doctor for anemia symptoms or slow blood loss in stool.
- If there is a history of heart disease in your family, consult your doctor before supplementing your diet with iron.

→

MINERALS

Pregnancy:
Pregnancy increases need. Check with doctor. During first 3 months of pregnancy, take only if your doctor prescribes it.

Breastfeeding:
- Supplements probably aren't necessary if you are healthy and eat a balanced diet. Consult your doctor.
- Your baby may need supplementation, especially premature infants. Consult your doctor.

Effect on lab tests:
Iron may cause abnormal results in serum bilirubin, serum calcium, serum iron, special radioactive studies of bones using technetium (Tc-99m-labeled agents) and stool studies for blood.

Storage:
- Store in cool, dry place away from direct light, but don't freeze.
- Store safely out of reach of children, with childproof cap. Iron tablets look like candy, and children have been known to overdose.
- Don't store in bathroom medicine cabinet. Heat and moisture may change the action of the mineral.

Others:
- Iron can accumulate to harmful levels (hemosiderosis) in patients with chronic kidney failure, Hodgkins disease or rheumatoid arthritis.
- Prolonged use in high doses can cause hemochromatosis (iron-storage disease), leading to bronze skin, diabetes, liver damage, impotence and heart problems.

 Overdose/Toxicity

Signs and symptoms:
- Early signs: Diarrhea with blood, severe nausea, abdominal pain, vomiting with blood
- Late signs: Weakness; collapse; pallor; blue lips, hands, fingernails; shallow breathing; convulsions; coma; weak, rapid heartbeat
- Too much iron may increase risk of cancer and coronary disease

What to do:
For symptoms of overdose:
Discontinue mineral and consult doctor. Also see *Adverse Reactions or Side Effects* section below.

For accidental overdose (such as child taking entire bottle): Dial 911 (emergency), 0 for operator or call your nearest Poison Control Center.

 Adverse Reactions or Side Effects

Reaction or effect	What to do
Abdominal pain	Discontinue. Call doctor immediately.
Black or gray stools (always)	Nothing.
Blood in stools	Seek emergency treatment.
Chest pain	Seek emergency treatment.
Drowsiness	Discontinue. Call doctor when convenient.
Stained tooth (with liquid forms)	Mix with water or juice to lessen effect. Brush teeth with baking soda or hydrogen peroxide to help remove stain.
Throat pain	Discontinue. Call doctor immediately.

Interaction with Medicine, Minerals or Vitamins

Interacts with	Combined effect
Allopurinol	May cause excess iron storage in liver.
Antacids	Causes poor iron absorption.
Calcium	Combination necessary for efficient calcium absorption.
Cholestyramine	Decreases iron effect.
Copper	Assists in copper absorption.
Iron supplements (other)	May cause excess iron storage in liver.
Pancreatin	Decreases iron absorption.
Penicillamine	Decreases penicillamine effect.
Sulfasalazine	Decreases iron effect.
Tetracyclines	Decreases tetracycline effect. Take iron 3 hours before or 2 hours after taking tetracycline.
Vitamin C	Increases iron effect. Necessary for red-blood-cell and hemoglobin formation.
Vitamin E	Decreases iron absorption.
Zinc (large doses)	Decreases iron absorption.

Interaction with Other Substances

Alcohol increases iron utilization and may cause organ damage. Avoid or use in moderation.

Food and beverages:
- Milk, cheese, yogurt and eggs decrease iron absorption.
- Tea decreases iron absorption.
- Coffee decreases iron absorption.
- Spinach decreases iron absorption.
- Bran, whole-grain breads and cereals decrease iron absorption.

Lab Tests to Detect Deficiency

- Red-blood-cell count
- Microscopic exam of red blood cells
- Serum iron, total iron-binding capacity
- Hemoglobin, low hematocrit determinations
- Serum ferritin

MINERALS

Magnesium

Basic Information

- Available from natural sources? Yes
- Available from synthetic sources? No
- Prescription required? Yes, for some forms
- *Optimal Intake,* see pages 182–183

Natural Sources

Almonds	Herring
Avocados	Leafy, green vegetables
Bananas	Mackerel
Bluefish	Molasses
Carp	Nuts
Cod	Ocean perch
Collards, beet greens	Shrimp
Dairy products	Swordfish
Flounder	Wheat germ
Halibut	Whole-wheat bread

Benefits

- Aids bone growth
- Aids function of nerves and muscles, including regulation of normal heart rhythm
- Conducts nerve impulses
- Works as laxative in large doses
- Acts as antacid in small doses
- Strengthens tooth enamel

Possible Additional Benefits

- May help reduce the effects of lead poisoning
- May reduce kidney stones
- May be used to treat heart disease

Who May Benefit from Additional Amounts?

- Anyone with inadequate caloric or dietary intake or increased nutritional requirements
- Those who abuse alcohol or other drugs
- People with a chronic wasting illness
- Anyone who has recently undergone surgery
- Anyone suffering with vomiting or diarrhea
- With medical supervision, may supplement treatment of those with acute myocardial infarction, cardiac surgery, digitalis toxicity and congestive heart failure

Deficiency Symptoms

Following symptoms occur rarely:
- Muscle contractions
- Convulsions
- Confusion, delirium, memory and concentration difficulties
- Irritability
- Nervousness
- Skin problems
- Hardening of soft tissues
- Hypertension
- Arrhythmia

Usage Information

What this mineral does:
- Activates essential enzymes
- Affects metabolism of proteins and nucleic acids
- Helps transport sodium and potassium across cell membranes
- Influences calcium levels inside cells
- Aids muscle contractions

Available as:
- Tablets, capsules, extended-release: Swallow whole with a full glass of liquid. Don't chew or crush. Take with or 1 to 1-1/2 hours after meals unless otherwise directed by your doctor.
- Liquid or powder: Follow manu-facturer's instructions. Swallow with *at least* one full glass of liquid. Drink plenty of fluids throughout the day.
- Magnesium is a constituent of many multivitamin/mineral preparations.
- Injectable forms are administered by a doctor or nurse.

Warnings and Precautions

Don't take if you have:
- Kidney failure
- Heart block (unless you have a pacemaker)
- Had an ileostomy

Consult your doctor if you have:
- Chronic constipation, colitis, diarrhea
- Symptoms of appendicitis
- Stomach or intestinal bleeding

Over 55:
Adverse reactions and side effects are more likely.

Pregnancy:
Risk to fetus. Don't use.

Breastfeeding:
Avoid magnesium except under advice of your physician.

Effect on lab tests:
• Inaccurate test for stomach-acid secretion
• May increase or decrease serum-phosphate concentrations
• May decrease serum and urine pH

Storage:
• Store in cool, dry place away from direct light, but don't freeze.
• Store safely out of reach of children.
• Don't store in bathroom medicine cabinet. Heat and moisture may change the action of the mineral.

Others:
• Chronic kidney disease causes body to retain excess magnesium.
• Adverse reactions, side effects and interactions with medicines, vitamins or minerals occur only rarely when you take too much magnesium for too long or if you have kidney disease.

Overdose/Toxicity

Signs and symptoms:
Severe nausea and vomiting, extremely low blood pressure, extreme muscle weakness, difficulty breathing, heartbeat irregularity.

What to do:
For symptoms of overdose:
Discontinue mineral and consult doctor immediately. Also see *Adverse Reactions or Side Effects* section below.

For accidental overdose (such as child taking entire bottle): Dial 911 (emergency), 0 for operator or call your nearest Poison Control Center.

Adverse Reactions or Side Effects

Reaction or effect	What to do
Abdominal pain	Discontinue. Call doctor immediately.
Appetite loss	Discontinue. Call doctor when convenient.
Diarrhea	Discontinue. Call doctor when convenient.
Irregular heartbeat	Seek emergency treatment.
Mood changes or mental changes	Discontinue. Call doctor when convenient.
Nausea	Discontinue. Call doctor when convenient.
Tiredness or weakness	Discontinue. Call doctor when convenient.
Urination discomfort	Discontinue. Call doctor when convenient.
Vomiting	Discontinue. Call doctor immediately.

Interaction with Medicine, Minerals or Vitamins

Interacts with	Combined effect
Antibiotics (some)	Decreases magnesium levels.
Cellulose sodium phosphate	Decreases magnesium effect. Take 1 or more hours apart.
Diuretics (some)	Decreases magnesium level.
Ketoconazole	Reduces absorption of ketoconazole. Take 2 hours apart.
Mecamylamine	May slow urinary excretion of mecamylamine. Avoid combination
Tetracycline	Decreases absorption of tetracycline.
Vitamin D	May raise magnesium level too high.

MINERALS

→

Lab Tests to Detect Deficiency

Serum magnesium

Manganese

Basic Information

- Available from natural sources? Yes
- Available from synthetic sources? Yes
- Prescription required? Yes, for some forms
- *Optimal Intake, see pages 182–183*

Natural Sources

Beans, dried	Oatmeal
Blue- and	Peanuts
blackberries	Peas
Bran	Pecans
Buckwheat	Seaweed
Carrots	Spinach
Chestnuts	Tea
Hazelnuts	Whole grains
(filberts)	

Benefits

- Promotes normal growth and development
- Helps many enzymes generate energy
- Aids in carbohydrate metabolism
- Promotes nerve function
- Aids in formation of connective tissue
- Involved in antioxidation process

Possible Additional Benefits

- May reduce asthmatic symptoms
- May enhance fertility
- May promote glucose transport

Who May Benefit from Additional Amounts?

Anyone with inadequate caloric or nutritional dietary intake or increased nutritional requirements

Deficiency Symptoms

Note: Deficiencies are extremely rare because manganese is widely available in the food supply and requirements are very small.

- Abnormal growth and development of children
- No proven symptoms caused by manganese deficiency in adults

Usage Information

What this mineral does:

- Manganese is concentrated in the cells of the pituitary gland, liver, pancreas, kidney and bone. It stimulates production of cholesterol

by the liver and is a cofactor (see Glossary) in many enzymes.
- Manganese works with vitamin K to promote blood clotting.

Miscellaneous information:
- Manganese is abundant in many foods.
- Manganese and magnesium are *not* related!

Available as:
- Capsules: Swallow whole with a full glass of liquid. Don't chew or crush. Take with food or immediately after eating to decrease stomach irritation.
- Manganese is a constituent of many multivitamin/mineral preparations.
- Injection: administered by a doctor or nurse.

 Warnings and Precautions

Don't take if you:
Are healthy and eat well.

Consult your doctor if you have:
- Liver disease
- Iron deficiency

Pregnancy:
Don't take supplements that contain manganese unless prescribed by your doctor.

Breastfeeding:
Don't take supplements that contain manganese unless prescribed by your doctor.

Effect on lab tests:
Excess manganese can reduce serum iron.

Storage:
- Store in cool, dry place away from direct light, but don't freeze.
- Store safely out of reach of children.
- Don't store in bathroom medicine cabinet. Heat and moisture may change the action of the mineral.

Others:
Check with your industrial health office if you are a miner or industrial worker to make sure your work environment does not contain toxic amounts of manganese.

 Overdose/Toxicity

Signs and symptoms:
Delusions, hallucinations, insomnia, depression, impotence

What to do:
For symptoms of overdose:
Discontinue mineral and consult doctor. Also see *Adverse Reactions or Side Effects* section below.

For accidental overdose (such as child taking entire bottle): Dial 911 (emergency), 0 for operator or call your nearest Poison Control Center.

 Adverse Reactions or Side Effects

Reaction or effect	What to do
Appetite loss	Discontinue. Call doctor when convenient.
Breathing problems	Seek emergency treatment.
Headaches	Discontinue. Call doctor when convenient.
Unusual tiredness	Discontinue. Call doctor when convenient.

Interaction with Medicine, Minerals or Vitamins

Interacts with	Combined effect
Calcium (from food or supplements)	May decrease manganese absorption when taken in large doses.
Iron (from food or supplements)	Excess manganese interferes with iron absorption and can lead to iron-deficiency anemia.
Magnesium (from food or supplements)	May decrease manganese absorption when taken in large doses.
Oral contraceptives	Decreases manganese in blood.
Phosphate (from food or supplements)	When taken in large doses, may decrease manganese absorption.

 Lab Tests to Detect Deficiency

Serum manganese

Molybdenum

 Basic Information

- Available from natural sources? Yes
- Available from synthetic sources? No
- Prescription required? Yes, for some forms
- *Optimal Intake,* see pages 182–183

 Natural Sources

Beans
Cereal grains, whole grains
Dark green, leafy vegetables
Lean meats
Organ meats (liver, kidney, sweetbreads)
Peas and other legumes
Note: The dietary concentration of molybdenum may vary according to the status of the soil in which grains and vegetables are raised. Deficiencies are extremely rare.

 Benefits

- Promotes normal growth and development
- Is a component of xanthine oxidase, an enzyme involved in converting nucleic acid to uric acid, a waste product eliminated in the urine

 Possible Additional Benefits

- May protect teeth
- May enhance iron absorption

 Who May Benefit from Additional Amounts?

- Anyone with inadequate caloric or nutritional dietary intake or increased nutritional requirements
- People with recent severe burns or injuries

- Extremely ill people who must be fed intravenously or by nasogastric tube

Deficiency Symptoms

No symptoms in humans. Deficiency is rare and occurs only in conjunction with other disorders.

Usage Information

What this mineral does:
- Becomes a part of bones, liver, kidney
- Forms part of the enzyme system of xanthine oxidase

Miscellaneous information:
A balanced diet provides all the molybdenum that is necessary in a healthy child or adult.

Available as:
- Capsules: Swallow whole with a full glass of liquid. Don't chew or crush. Take with or 1 to 1-1/2 hours after meals unless otherwise directed by your doctor.
- Injectable forms are administered by a doctor or nurse.
- Molybdenum is a constituent of many multivitamin/mineral preparations.

Warnings and Precautions

Don't take if you:
No problems are expected at 0.15 to 0.5mg/day. Don't take higher doses without a doctor's prescription.

Consult your doctor if you have:
- High levels of uric acid
- Gout
- Copper deficiency
- Kidney or liver disease

Pregnancy:
Don't take.

Breastfeeding:
Don't take.

Effect on lab tests:
Excess molybdenum causes serum-copper level to drop.

Storage:
- Store in cool, dry place away from direct light, but don't freeze.
- Store safely out of reach of children.
- Don't store in bathroom medicine cabinet. Heat and moisture may change the action of the mineral.

Overdose/Toxicity

Signs and symptoms:
Gout and a goutlike syndrome can be produced by massive intake (10 to 15mg/day). Moderate excess (up to 0.54mg/day) can cause excess loss of copper in urine.

What to do:
For symptoms of overdose:
Discontinue mineral and consult doctor.

For accidental overdose (such as child taking entire bottle): Dial 911 (emergency), 0 for operator or call your nearest Poison Control Center.

MINERALS

→

Adverse Reactions or Side Effects

None are expected.

Lab Tests to Detect Deficiency

None are available, except for experimental purposes.

Interaction with Medicine, Minerals or Vitamins

Interacts with	Combined effect
Copper	Maintains appropriate ratio of molybdenum and copper in body. With excess molybdenum, copper level drops. With excess copper, molybdenum level drops.
Sulfur	Increased sulfur intake causes decline in molybdenum concentration.

Phosphorus

Basic Information

- Available from natural sources? Yes
- Available from synthetic sources? No
- Prescription required? Yes, for medical purposes
- *Optimal Intake,* see pags 182–183

Natural Sources

Almonds
Beans, dried
Calf liver
Cheese, cheddar
Cheese, pasteurized
Eggs
Fish
Milk
Milk products
Peanuts
Peas
Poultry
Pumpkin seeds
Red meat
Sardines, canned
Scallops
Soda
Soybeans
Sunflower seeds
Tuna
Whole-grain products

Benefits

- Builds strong bones and teeth (with calcium)
- Promotes metabolism
- Promotes growth, maintenance and repair of all body tissues
- Buffers body fluids for acid-base balance
- Acidifies urine and reduces possibility of kidney stones

Possible Additional Benefits

None are known.

Who May Benefit from Additional Amounts?

- Anyone suffering prolonged vomiting
- Those with inadequate caloric or dietary intake or increased nutritional requirements
- Those who take excessive amounts of antacid
- People with a chronic wasting illness
- Those under excess stress for long periods
- Anyone who has recently undergone surgery
- Those with liver disease
- People with hyperparathyroidism
- Alcoholics

Deficiency Symptoms

- Bone pain
- Loss of appetite
- Weakness
- Easily broken bones

Usage Information

What this mineral does:
- Necessary for utilization of many B-complex vitamins
- An important constituent of all fats, proteins, carbohydrates and many enzymes

Available as:
- Tablets: Swallow whole with a full glass of liquid. Don't chew or crush. Take with or 1 to 1-1/2 hours after meals unless otherwise directed by your doctor.
- Capsules for oral solution: Empty contents into at least 1/2 glass of water or other liquid. Don't swallow filled capsule. Take with or 1 to 1-1/2 hours after meals unless otherwise directed by your doctor.
- Oral solution: Dilute in at least 1/2 glass of water or other liquid. Take with or 1 to 1-1/2 hours after meals unless otherwise directed by your doctor.
- Phosphorus is a constituent of many multivitamin/mineral preparations.

Warnings and Precautions

Don't take if you have:
- Kidney disease
- Kidney stones, and analysis has shown their composition to be magnesium ammonium phosphate

Consult your doctor if you have:
- Hypoparathyroidism
- Osteomalacia
- Acute pancreatitis
- Chronic kidney disease
- Rickets
- Adrenal insufficiency (Addison's disease)
- Dehydration
- Severe burns
- Heart disease
- Edema
- High blood pressure
- Toxemia of pregnancy

Pregnancy:
Take under doctor's supervision only. Don't take megadoses.

Breastfeeding:
Take under doctor's supervision only. Don't take megadoses.

MINERALS

Effect on lab tests:
May show false decrease in bone uptake in technetium-labeled diagnostic-imaging tests

Storage:
- Store in cool, dry place away from direct light, but don't freeze.
- Store safely out of reach of children.
- Don't store in bathroom medicine cabinet. Heat and moisture may change the action of the mineral.

Overdose/Toxicity

Signs and symptoms:
- Seizures, heartbeat irregularities, shortness of breath
- May increase calcium excretion and lead to osteoporosis

What to do:
For symptoms of overdose:
Discontinue mineral and seek emergency treatment. Also see *Adverse Reactions or Side Effects* section below.

For accidental overdose (such as child taking entire bottle): Dial 911 (emergency), 0 for operator or call your nearest Poison Control Center.

Adverse Reactions or Side Effects

Reaction or effect	What to do
Abdominal pain	Discontinue. Call doctor immediately.
Bone or joint pain	Discontinue. Call doctor immediately.
Breathing problems	Discontinue. Call doctor immediately.
Confusion	Discontinue. Call doctor immediately.
Convulsions	Discontinue. Call doctor immediately.
Decreased volume of urine in one day	Seek emergency treatment.
Fast, slow or irregular heartbeat	Discontinue. Call doctor immediately.
Headaches	Discontinue. Call doctor immediately.
Muscle cramps	Discontinue. Call doctor when convenient.
Numbness or tingling in hands or feet	Discontinue. Call doctor when convenient.
Tremor	Discontinue. Call doctor immediately.
Unusual thirst	Discontinue. Call doctor when convenient.

Interaction with Medicine, Minerals or Vitamins

Interacts with	Combined effect
Anabolic steroids	Increases risk of edema.
Antacids with aluminum or magnesium	May prevent absorption of phosphorus.
Calcium-containing supplements and antacids	May decrease phosphorus absorption.
Captopril	Increases risk of too much potassium (hyperkalemia).
Corticosteroids	Decreases phosphorus absorption.
Cortisone drugs or ACTH	Increases serum sodium.
Digitalis preparations	Increases risk of too much potassium (hyperkalemia).
Dilantin	May decrease phosphorus absorption.
Enalapril	Increases risk of too much potassium (hyperkalemia).
Iron supplements	Do not take within 1 to 2 hours of taking potassium phosphate as it may interfere with iron supplement.
Salicylates	May increase plasma concentration of salicylates.

Testosterone	Increases risk of edema.
Vitamin D	Enhances phosphorus absorption but may increase chance of too much phosphorus in blood and body cells.

Interaction with Other Substances

Alcohol decreases available phosphorus for vital body functions.

Lab Tests to Detect Deficiency

Serum phosphorus

Potassium

Basic Information

Potassium chloride is the most common form. This combination is also called *trikates*.

- Available from natural sources? Yes
- Available from synthetic sources? Yes
- Prescription required? Yes, for some forms
- *Optimal Intake*, see pages 182–183

Natural Sources

Asparagus	Molasses
Avocados	Nuts
Bananas	Parsnips
Beans	Peas (fresh)
Cantaloupe	Potatoes
Carrots	Raisins
Chard	Salt substitute
Citrus fruit	Sardines, canned
Juices (grapefruit, tomato, orange)	Spinach, fresh
Milk	Whole-grain cereal

Benefits

- Promotes regular heartbeat
- Promotes normal muscle contraction
- Helps prevent high blood pressure
- Regulates transfer of nutrients to cells
- Maintains water balance in body tissues and cells
- Preserves or restores normal function of nerve cells, heart cells, skeletal-muscle cells, kidneys, stomach-juice secretion
- Treats potassium deficiency from illness or taking diuretics (water pills), cortisone drugs or digitalis preparations

Possible Additional Benefits

- May cure alcoholism
- May cure acne
- Possible allergy cure
- Possible heart disease cure
- May help heal burns

Who May Benefit from Additional Amounts?

- People who take diuretics, cortisone drugs or digitalis preparations
- Anyone with inadequate caloric or nutritional dietary intake or increased nutritional requirements
- People over 55 years old
- Pregnant or breastfeeding women
- Women taking oral contraceptives
- People who abuse alcohol, tobacco or other drugs
- People with a chronic wasting illness
- Those under excess stress for long periods
- Anyone who has recently undergone surgery
- Athletes and workers who participate in vigorous physical activities, especially when endurance is an important aspect of the activity
- Those with part of the gastrointestinal tract surgically removed
- People with malabsorption disorders (See Glossary)
- Those with recent severe burns or injuries
- Vegetarians

Deficiency Symptoms

- Hypokalemia
- Weakness, paralysis
- Low blood pressure
- Irregular or rapid heartbeat that can lead to cardiac arrest and death

Usage Information

What this mineral does:

Potassium is the predominant positive electrolyte (see Glossary) in body cells. An enzyme (adenosine triphosphatase) controls the flow of potassium and sodium into and out of cells to maintain normal function of the heart, brain, skeletal muscles and kidney, and to maintain acid-base balance.

Miscellaneous information:

Avoid cooking food in large amounts of water.

Available as:

- Oral solution: Dilute in at least 1/2 glass of water or other liquid. Take with meals unless otherwise directed by your doctor.
- Potassium is not recommended for children.
- Some forms are available by generic name.

Warnings and Precautions

Don't take if you:

- Take potassium-sparing diuretics, such as spironolactone, triamterene or amiloride
- Are allergic to any potassium supplement
- Have kidney disease

Consult your doctor if you:

- Have Addison's disease
- Have diabetes
- Have heart disease
- Have intestinal blockage
- Have a stomach ulcer
- Take diuretics
- Take heart medicine
- Take laxatives or if you have chronic diarrhea
- Use salt substitutes or low-salt milk

Over 55:

- Observe dose schedule strictly; potassium balance is critical. Deviation above or below normal levels can have serious results.
- There is a greater risk of hyperkalemia.

Pregnancy:
No problems are expected. Consult your doctor.

Breastfeeding:
Studies are inconclusive on risk to infants. Consult your doctor about supplements.

Effect on lab tests:
- ECG and kidney function studies can be affected by too much or too little potassium.
- No effect is expected on blood studies, except serum-potassium levels.

Storage:
- Store in cool, dry place away from direct light, but don't freeze.
- Store safely out of reach of children.
- Don't store in bathroom medicine cabinet. Heat and moisture may change the action of the mineral

Others:
Take with food.

 Overdose/Toxicity

Signs and symptoms:
Irregular or fast heartbeat, paralysis of arms and legs, blood-pressure drop, convulsions, coma, cardiac arrest

What to do:
For symptoms of overdose:
Discontinue mineral and consult doctor immediately. Also see *Adverse Reactions or Side Effects* section below.

For accidental overdose (such as child taking entire bottle): Dial 911 (emergency), 0 for operator or call your nearest Poison Control Center. If person's heart has stopped beating, render CPR until trained help arrives.

 Adverse Reactions or Side Effects

Reaction or effect	What to do
Black, tarry stool	Seek emergency treatment.
Bloody stool	Seek emergency treatment.
Breathing difficulty	Seek emergency treatment.
Confusion	Discontinue. Call doctor immediately.
Diarrhea	Discontinue. Call doctor immediately.
Extreme fatigue	Discontinue. Call doctor when convenient.
Heaviness in legs	Discontinue. Call doctor when convenient.
Irregular heartbeat	Seek emergency treatment.
Nausea	Discontinue. Call doctor when convenient.
Numbness in hands or feet	Discontinue. Call doctor when convenient.
Stomach discomfort	Discontinue. Call doctor when convenient.
Tingling in hands or feet	Discontinue. Call doctor when convenient.
Vomiting	Discontinue. Call doctor immediately.
Weakness	Discontinue. Call doctor immediately.

 Interaction with Medicine, Minerals or Vitamins

Interacts with	Combined effect
Amiloride	Causes dangerous rise in blood potassium.
Atropine	Increases possibility of intestinal ulcers, which may occur with oral potassium.
Belladonna	Increases possibility of intestinal ulcers, which may occur with oral potassium.

MINERALS

→

Calcium	Increases possibility of heartbeat irregularities.
Captopril	Increases chance of excessive amounts of potassium.
Cortisone	Decreases effect of potassium.
Digitalis preparations	May cause irregular heartbeat.
Enalapril	Increases chance of excessive amounts of potassium.
Laxatives	May decrease potassium effect.
Spironolactone	Increases blood potassium.
Triamterene	Increases blood potassium.
Vitamin B-12	Extended-release tablets may decrease vitamin B-12 absorption and increase vitamin B-12 requirements.

Alcohol intensifies gastrointestinal symptoms.

Cocaine may cause irregular heartbeat.

Marijuana may cause irregular heartbeat.

Beverages:
- Salty drinks, such as tomato juice and commercial thirst quenchers, cause increased fluid retention.
- Coffee decreases potassium absorption and intensifies gastrointestinal symptoms.
- Low-salt milk increases fluid retention.

Foods:
- Salty foods increase fluid retention.
- Sugar decreases potassium absorption.

Interaction with Other Substances

Tobacco decreases absorption. Smokers may require supplemental potassium.

Lab Tests to Detect Deficiency

- Serum-potassium determinations
- Serum creatinine
- Electrocardiograms
- Serum-pH determinations

Selenium

Basic Information

- Available from natural sources? Yes
- Available from synthetic sources? No
- Prescription required? No
- *Optimal Intake,* see pages 182–183

Natural Sources

Bran
Broccoli
Brown rice
Cabbage
Chicken
Garlic (grown in selenium-rich soil)
Kidney
Liver
Milk
Mushrooms
Nutritional yeast
Oatmeal
Onions
Seafood
Tuna
Whole-grain products

Note: The selenium content of food varies greatly because of the wide variability of this element in the soil. Foods grown in the southeastern United States are known to have lower selenium content.

Benefits

- Complements vitamin E as an efficient antioxidant (see Glossary)
- Promotes normal growth and development
- Functions as antioxidant itself
- Stimulates immune system
- Protects against prostate cancer

Possible Additional Benefits

- May protect against increased oxidation (see Glossary) associated with aging
- May protect against cardiovascular disease, strokes and heart attacks
- Potentially decreases platelet clumping in bloodstream and prevents clots at site of blood-vessel damage in heart and brain
- May protect against damage caused by tobacco smoking
- May be extremely strong antioxidant (see Glossary)
- May reduce cataract formation through antioxidation

Who May Benefit from Additional Amounts?

- Anyone with inadequate caloric or nutritional dietary intake or increased nutritional requirements
- People who live in areas where soil is selenium-deficient, such as China, New Zealand and central and southeastern United States (check with your local county agricultural agent)
- Anyone with celiac disease
- HIV/AIDS patients

Deficiency Symptoms

Selenium deficiency has resulted in cardiomyopathy and myocardial deaths in humans.

Usage Information

What this mineral does:
Selenium helps defend against damage from oxidation.

Miscellaneous information:
- Selenium should be part of a well-balanced vitamin and mineral regimen.
- Protection from human degenerative disorders has yet to be proved.
- Experimental studies are trying to prove that selenium plays a big part as an antioxidant (see Glossary) nutrient to help protect against damaging free radicals (see Glossary).
- Organic forms (from foods or brewer's yeast) are less toxic than inorganic sodium selenide.
- No one can be sure of the correct amount to be ingested each day. People who eat a balanced diet of food grown in the western United States probably get enough from food.

Available as:
- Tablets or capsules: Swallow whole with a full glass of liquid. Don't chew or crush. Take with or 1 to 1-1/2 hours after meals unless otherwise directed by your doctor.
- Selenium is a constituent of many multivitamin/mineral preparations.

MINERALS

Warnings and Precautions

Don't take if you:
Plan to use it on the scalp or skin for seborrheic dermatitis or dandruff if you have any inflammation or oozing.

Consult your doctor if you:
Plan to take more than the dose recommended by the manufacturer.

Over 55:
No problems are expected with usual doses.

Pregnancy:
No problems are expected with usual doses.

Breastfeeding:
No problems are expected with usual doses.

Storage:
• Store in cool, dry place away from direct light, but don't freeze.
• Store safely out of reach of children.
• Don't store in bathroom medicine cabinet. Heat and moisture may change the action of the mineral.

Others:
Workers at industrial sites that manufacture glass, pesticides, rubber, semiconductors, copper and film are at increased risk of developing toxic symptoms from inhalation, absorption through the skin and ingestion. These symptoms may include bronchial pneumonia, asthma, precipitous drop in blood pressure, red eyes, garlic odor on breath and in urine, headaches, metallic taste, nose and throat irritation, difficulty breathing, vomiting and weakness.

 ## Overdose/Toxicity

Signs and symptoms:
• Toxicity is unlikely to develop with organic selenium if you don't consume more than the regular dose recommended by the manufacturer.
• Individuals in industrial settings have been reported to suffer toxic symptoms of selenium overdoses, including liver disease and cardiomyopathy.
• Children reared in selenium-rich areas show a higher incidence of decayed, missing and filled teeth.
• Selenium is toxic in megadoses and may cause alopecia (hair loss), loss of nails, fatigue, nausea, vomiting, lesions and sour-milk breath.

What to do:
For symptoms of overdose:
Discontinue mineral and consult doctor. Also see *Adverse Reactions or Side Effects* section below.

For accidental overdose (such as child taking entire bottle): Dial 911 (emergency), 0 for operator or call your nearest Poison Control Center.

 ## Adverse Reactions or Side Effects

Reaction or effect	What to do
Dizziness and nausea, without other apparent cause	Discontinue. Call doctor immediately.
Fragile or black fingernails	Discontinue. Call doctor when convenient.
Persistent garlic odor on breath and skin	Discontinue. Call doctor when convenient.
Unusual dryness when used on scalp or skin	Discontinue. Call doctor when convenient.
Unusual hair loss or discoloration of hair	Discontinue. Call doctor when convenient.

Interaction with Medicine, Minerals or Vitamins

Interacts with	Combined effect
Vitamin C	May decrease selenium absorption if taken with an inorganic form of selenium.
Vitamin E	Prevents oxidation that might cause breakdown of body chemicals.

Lab Tests to Detect Deficiency

24-hour urine collection

MINERALS

Silicon

Basic Information

- Available from natural sources? Yes
- Available from synthetic sources? Yes
- Prescription required? No

Natural Sources

Apples	Legumes
Beets	Root vegetables
Brown rice	Soybeans
Horsetail	Whole grains

Benefits

Essential for collagen formation

Possible Additional Benefits

- May aid early stages of calcium absorption
- May boost immune system
- May prevent osteoporosis
- May improve nails, skin and hair
- May reduce risk of cardiovascular disease
- May help reduce blood pressure

Who May Benefit from Additional Amounts?

Unknown

Deficiency Symptoms

Deficiency is not known because silicon is available in so many foods.

Usage Information

What this mineral does:

- Plays a role in bone growth
- Strengthens blood vessels, cartilage and tendons

Miscellaneous information:

- Most of the silicon present in the body is found in connective tissue.
- Studies on chicks showed that silicon deficiency causes skull, bone and joint abnormalities.

Available as:

- Liquid: Take as directed by manufacturer or your doctor.
- Tablet: Take as directed by manufacturer or your doctor.

Warnings and Precautions

Pregnancy:
Do not take.

Breastfeeding:
Do not take.

Storage:
- Store in cool, dry place away from direct light, but don't freeze.
- Store safely out of reach of children.
- Don't store in bathroom medicine cabinet. Heat and moisture may change the action of the mineral.

Overdose/Toxicity

What to do:
For symptoms of overdose:
Discontinue mineral and consult doctor immediately.

For accidental overdose (such as child taking entire bottle): Dial 911 (emergency), 0 for operator or call your nearest Poison Control Center.

Adverse Reactions or Side Effects

None are known.

Interaction with Medicine, Minerals or Vitamins

Interacts with	Combined effect
Aluminum	Counteracts effect of aluminum.
Boron	Helps body utilize silicon.
Calcium	Helps body utilize silicon.
Magnesium	Helps body utilize silicon.
Manganese	Helps body utilize silicon.
Potassium	Helps body utilize silicon.

Lab Tests to Detect Deficiency

No existing tests because deficiency doesn't occur.

Sodium

Basic Information

- Available from natural sources? Yes
- Available from synthetic sources? No
- Prescription required? No
- *Optimal Intake,* see pages 182–183

Natural Sources

Bacon
Beef, dried
    and fresh
Bread
Butter
Clams
Green beans
Ham
Margarine
Milk

Olives
Pickles
Processed meat
Salted nuts,
    snack foods
Sardines, canned
Table salt (chief
    source of sodium)
Tomatoes, canned

Note: In most commercially canned vegetables and processed foods, salt is added to improve taste. "Highly processed" foods (also high in sodium) include soups, bouillon, pickles, potato chips, snack foods and ham.

Benefits

- Helps regulate water balance in body
- Plays a crucial role in maintaining normal blood pressure
- Aids muscle contraction and nerve transmission
- Regulates body's acid-base balance

Possible Additional Benefits

Low-sodium diets appear to reduce high blood pressure in some individuals.

Who May Benefit from Additional Amounts?

- Anyone who suffers prolonged loss of body fluids from vomiting or diarrhea
- Those with Addison's disease
- Those who drink water excessively for prolonged periods (usually a psychiatric condition)
- People who suffer some types of cancer of the adrenal glands
- Those who sweat excessively due to heavy exercise or workload
- People who use diuretics (generally low-sodium diet is also prescribed to prevent fluid retention)
- Those with chronic kidney disease

Deficiency Symptoms

- Muscle and stomach cramps
- Nausea

- Fatigue
- Mental apathy
- Muscle twitching and cramping (usually in legs)
- Appetite loss

In severe cases:
Shock resulting from a decrease in blood pressure

Usage Information

What this mineral does:
As an electrolyte (see Glossary), sodium is present in all body cells. Its most important function is to regulate the balance of water inside and outside cells.

Miscellaneous information:
- We consume most of our sodium as sodium chloride—ordinary table salt.
- The most common problem with sodium in a healthy person is too much, rather than too little. A typical diet contains 3,000 to 12,000mg of sodium a day. Recommended intake is 2,400mg/day.
- Excessive amounts of sodium can be a major factor in the development of high blood pressure. Decreasing sodium intake helps control high blood pressure.
- There is speculation that the relationship between sodium intake and high blood pressure is actually more closely related to the sodium-potassium ratio. Certain people are "sodium sensitive" and will have lower blood pressure in response to a low-sodium diet.

Available as:
Sodium-chloride tablets, but these may cause stomach distress and an overload on the kidneys.

MINERALS

→

Warnings and Precautions

Don't take if you have:
- Congestive heart failure
- Hepatic cirrhosis
- Hypertension
- Edema from any cause
- A family history of high blood pressure

Consult your doctor if you have:
- Any heart or blood-vessel disease
- Bleeding problems
- Epilepsy
- Kidney disease

Over 55:
No problems are expected in healthy individuals.

Pregnancy:
Dietary restriction of sodium in healthy women during pregnancy is not recommended.

Breastfeeding:
Dietary restriction of sodium in healthy women during lactation is not recommended.

Storage:
- Store in cool, dry place away from direct light, but don't freeze.
- Store safely out of reach of children.
- Don't store in bathroom medicine cabinet. Heat and moisture may change the action of the mineral.

Others:
- Too little sodium occurs almost entirely in people desperately ill with dehydration, recovering from recent surgery or after excessive sweating from heavy physical activity in a hot environment.

- Proper replacement of sodium deficiencies requires care by your doctor and frequent lab studies.

 ## Overdose/Toxicity

Signs and symptoms:
Tissue swelling (edema), stupor, coma

What to do:
For symptoms of overdose:
Discontinue mineral and consult doctor. Also see *Adverse Reactions or Side Effects* section below.

For accidental overdose (such as child taking entire bottle): Dial 911 (emergency), 0 for operator or call your nearest Poison Control Center.

 ## Adverse Reactions or Side Effects

Reaction or effect	What to do
With excessive amounts of sodium:	
Anxiety	Discontinue. Call doctor immediately.
Confusion	Discontinue. Call doctor immediately.
Edema	Discontinue. Call doctor immediately.
Nausea	Discontinue. Call doctor immediately.
Restlessness	Discontinue. Call doctor immediately.
Vomiting	Seek emergency treatment.
Weakness	Discontinue. Call doctor immediately.

 ## Interaction with Medicine, Minerals or Vitamins

None are expected.

Lab Tests to Detect Deficiency

Serum sodium

Sulfur

Basic Information

- Available from natural sources? Yes
- Available from synthetic sources? No
- Prescription required? No

Natural Sources

Beans, dried	Lean beef, meats
Eggs	Milk
Fish	Poultry
Garlic	Wheat germ

Benefits

- Plays a role in oxidation-reduction reactions (see Glossary)
- Aids bile secretion in liver
- Aids metabolism

Possible Additional Benefits

- May extend life span
- May protect against toxic substances
- May reduce arthritis symptoms
- Methyl sulfonyl methane has been used to treat allergies

Who May Benefit from Additional Amounts?

Supplements are probably not needed—no recorded deficiency states.

Deficiency Symptoms

No proven symptoms exist.

Usage Information

What this mineral does:
- Sulfur is part of the chemical structure of cysteine, methionine, taurine and glutathione.
- Sulfur aids treatment of aluminum, cadmium, mercury and lead poisoning.
- It is a component of biotin and B-1.

Available as:
A constituent of many multivitamin/mineral preparations.

Warnings and Precautions

Pregnancy:
No problems are expected.

Breastfeeding:
No problems are expected.

Storage:
- Store in cool, dry place away from direct light, but don't freeze.
- Store safely out of reach of children.
- Don't store in bathroom medicine cabinet. Heat and moisture may change the action of the mineral.

➔

MINERALS

Overdose/Toxicity

Signs and symptoms:
Unlikely to threaten life or cause significant symptoms.

What to do:
For symptoms of overdose:
Discontinue mineral and consult doctor.

For accidental overdose (such as child taking entire bottle): Dial 911 (emergency), 0 for operator or call your nearest Poison Control Center.

Adverse Reactions or Side Effects

None are known.

Interaction with Medicine, Minerals or Vitamins

None are known.

Interaction with Other Substances

Tobacco decreases absorption. Smokers may require supplemental sulfur.

Lab Tests to Detect Deficiency

None are available, except for experimental purposes.

Vanadium

Basic Information

• Available from natural sources? Yes
• Available from synthetic sources? No
• Prescription required? No

Natural Sources

Cereals	Mushrooms
Dill	Parsley
Fish/seafood	Soy
Liver	

Benefits

Plays role in metabolism of bones and teeth

Possible Additional Benefits

May help prevent heart attacks

Who May Benefit from Additional Amounts?

Supplements are probably not needed—no recorded deficiency states.

 ## Deficiency Symptoms

A vanadium-deficient diet fed to laboratory animals resulted in impaired reproductive ability and increased infant mortality.

 ## Usage Information

What this mineral does:
- Unknown effect in humans, but believed to be essential
- May be a part of cholesterol metabolism as well as hormone production

Miscellaneous information:
- Even the most nutritionally inadequate diet contains sufficient quantities to prevent a deficiency.
- Research is being conducted regarding the role of vanadium intake and thyroid.

Available as:
- Capsules: Swallow whole with a full glass of liquid. Don't chew or crush. Take with or 1 to 1-1/2 hours after meals unless otherwise directed by your doctor.
- Vanadium is a constituent of many multivitamin/mineral preparations.

 ## Warnings and Precautions

Pregnancy:
No problems are expected.

Breastfeeding:
No problems are expected.

Storage:
- Store in cool, dry place away from direct light, but don't freeze.
- Store safely out of reach of children.
- Don't store in bathroom medicine cabinet. Heat and moisture may change the action of the mineral.

 ## Overdose/Toxicity

Signs and symptoms:
Toxicity would likely affect kidney, liver or spleen function, and bone marrow.

What to do:
For symptoms of overdose:
Discontinue mineral and consult doctor.

For accidental overdose (such as child taking entire bottle): Dial 911 (emergency), 0 for operator or call your nearest Poison Control Center.

 ## Adverse Reactions or Side Effects

None are expected.

MINERALS

Interaction with Medicine, Minerals or Vitamins

Interacts with	Combined effect
Chromium	Chromium and vanadium may interfere with each other.

Lab Tests to Detect Deficiency

None are available, except for experimental purposes.

Zinc

Basic Information

- Available from natural sources? Yes
- Available from synthetic sources? No
- Prescription required? No
- *Optimal Intake,* see pages 182–183

Natural Sources

Beef, lean	Pork
Chicken heart	Sesame seeds
Egg yolk	Soybeans
Fish	Sunflower seeds
Herring	Turkey
Lamb	Wheat bran
Maple syrup	Wheat germ
Milk	Whole-grain
Molasses,	products
blackstrap	Yeast
Oysters	

Benefits

- Functions in antioxidant reactions (see Glossary)
- Maintains normal taste and sense of smell
- Promotes normal growth and development
- Treats burns and aids wound healing
- Promotes normal fetal growth
- Helps synthesize DNA and RNA
- Promotes cell division, repair and growth
- Maintains normal level of vitamin A in blood
- Boosts immunity in zinc-deficient people
- Treats Wilson's disease

Possible Additional Benefits

- May promote normal fertility
- May increase attention span and improve short-term memory

Who May Benefit from Additional Amounts?

- Anyone with inadequate caloric or nutritional dietary intake or increased nutritional requirements, such as vegetarians
- Preschool children with inadequate diet
- People over 55 years old

- Those who abuse alcohol or other drugs
- People with a chronic wasting illness
- Those under excess stress for long periods
- Anyone who has recently undergone surgery
- People with recent severe burns or injuries
- Anyone taking diuretics (water pills) for any reason, such as high blood pressure, congestive heart failure, liver disease
- Those who live in areas where soil is deficient in zinc
- Babies born with acrodermatitis enteropathica
- Anyone with Crohn's or celiac disease
- People with chronic diarrhea

Deficiency Symptoms

Moderate deficiency:
- Loss of taste and smell
- Slow growth in children
- Alopecia
- Rashes
- Multiple skin lesions
- Glossitis (See Glossary)
- Stomatitis (See Glossary)
- Blepharitis (See Glossary)
- Paronychia (See Glossary)
- Sterility
- Low sperm count
- Delayed wound healing

Serious deficiency:
- Delayed bone maturation
- Enlarged spleen or liver
- Decreased size of testicles
- Testicular function less than normal
- Decreased growth or dwarfism
- Problems relating to the eye such as optic neuritis, poor color discrimination, cataract formation

Usage Information

What this mineral does:
Zinc is a part of the molecular structure of 80 or more known enzymes. These particular enzymes work with red blood cells to move carbon dioxide from tissues to lungs.

Miscellaneous information:
- Zinc toxicity from inhalation is rare but can occur in the following industries and occupations: alloy manufacturing, brass foundry, bronze foundry, electric-fuse manufacturing, gas welding, electroplating, galvanizing, paint manufacturing, metal cutting, metal spraying, rubber manufacturing, roof manufacturing and zinc manufacturing.
- If you take zinc supplements, take with food to decrease gastric irritation.
- If taking zinc long term, also take 2 to 3mg/day of copper.
- Large doses of zinc may decrease HDL (see Glossary) cholesterol levels.

Available as:
- Tablets: Swallow whole with a full glass of liquid. Don't chew or crush. Take with or up to 1 to 1-1/2 hours after meals unless otherwise directed by your doctor.
- Zinc is a constituent of many multivitamin/mineral preparations.

Warnings and Precautions

Don't take if you have:
Stomach or duodenal ulcers.

Consult your doctor if you:
- Plan to take more than the manufacturer's recommended dose

➡

- Plan to take any calcium supplement or tetracycline drugs (zinc may interfere with absorption of these medicines)

Over 55:
Deficiency is more likely.

Pregnancy:
- Many diets are marginally low in zinc and may not supply the zinc required during pregnancy. Ask your doctor about supplementation.
- Overconsumption is dangerous and can lead to premature labor or stillbirth.
- Deficiency may be a factor in toxemia and could also be a factor in low-birthweight babies. Ask your doctor for advice.
- Zinc treats nausea in pregnancy.

Breastfeeding:
Some diets are marginally low in zinc and may not supply the zinc required while breastfeeding. Ask your doctor about supplementation.

Effect on lab tests:
- Zinc decreases high-density lipoprotein levels in young males. High-density lipoproteins decrease risk of coronary-artery disease.
- High doses decrease copper in blood.

Storage:
- Store in cool, dry place away from direct light, but don't freeze.
- Store safely out of reach of children.
- Don't store in bathroom medicine cabinet. Heat and moisture may change the action of the mineral.

Overdose/Toxicity

Signs and symptoms:
- Toxicity at RDA doses is highly unlikely. Toxic symptoms are extremes of the *Adverse Reactions or Side Effects* listed below.

- Overdose produces drowsiness, lethargy, lightheadedness, difficulty writing, staggering gait, restlessness and excessive vomiting leading to dehydration.

What to do:
For symptoms of overdose:
Discontinue mineral and consult doctor. Also see *Adverse Reactions or Side Effects* section below.

For accidental overdose (such as child taking entire bottle): Dial 911 (emergency), 0 for operator or call your nearest Poison Control Center.

Adverse Reactions or Side Effects

Reaction or effect	What to do
Abdominal pain	Seek emergency treatment.
Abnormal bleeding	Seek emergency treatment.
Diarrhea (mild)	Discontinue. Call doctor when convenient.
Gastric ulceration (burning pain in upper chest relieved by food or antacid)	Discontinue. Call doctor immediately.
Nausea or vomiting	Discontinue. Call doctor immediately.

Interaction with Medicine, Minerals or Vitamins

Interacts with	Combined effect
Calcium	Interferes with calcium absorption.
Copper	Decreases absorption of copper. Large or long-term doses of zinc must be taken to produce this effect.
Cortisone drugs	May interfere with lab tests measuring zinc.
Diuretics	Increases zinc excretion. Greater amounts of zinc required.

Iron	Decreases absorption of iron. Large doses of zinc must be taken to produce this effect.
Oral contraceptives	Lowers zinc blood levels.
Tetracycline	Decreases amount of tetracycline absorbed into bloodstream. Zinc and tetracycline should not be mixed. Take at least 2 hours apart.
Vitamin A	Assists in absorption of vitamin A.

 ## Interaction with Other Substances

Alcohol, even in moderate amounts, can increase the excretion of zinc in urine and can impair the body's ability to combine zinc into its proper enzyme combinations in the liver.

Beverages: Do not drink coffee at the same time as taking zinc because it may decrease zinc absorption.

 ## Lab Tests to Detect Deficiency

Serum zinc (by atomic absorption spectroscopy)

MINERALS

Vitamins

Vitamin is a general term for unrelated organic compounds. Organic compounds all contain the carbon atom. Vitamins occur in small amounts in many foods and are widely dispersed in our food supply.

Vitamins are necessary for normal metabolic functioning of the body. They form a part of enzymes to help complete chemical reactions in the body and are components of hormones. Vitamins may make solutions only in water (water-soluble) or only in fatty liquids (fat-soluble). Without vitamins, life-threatening deficiency diseases can occur, including scurvy from a vitamin-C deficiency, or even pellagra (see Glossary) from a niacin deficiency. Deficiency is rare in the United States because of the abundance of food. Therefore, in recent times, our attention has shifted from treating deficiency to optimizing health with vitamins. Vitamins present in foods are considered *natural* vitamins; those created in a laboratory are considered *synthetic.*

Vitamin A (Beta-carotene, Retinol)

Basic Information

Beta-carotene is a previtamin-A compound found in plants. The body converts beta-carotene to vitamin A.

Retinol comes from animal products such as liver, egg yolk, cheese and milk.

- Available from natural sources? Yes
- Available from synthetic sources? Yes
- Prescription required? No
- Fat-soluble
- *Optimal Intake,* see pages 182–183

Natural Sources

Apricots, fresh	Liver
Asparagus	Milk
Broccoli	Mustard greens
Cantaloupe	Pumpkin
Carrots	Spinach
Eggs	Squash, winter
Endive, raw	Sweet potatoes
Kale	Tomatoes
Leaf lettuce	Watermelon

Benefits

- Aids in treatment of some eye disorders, including prevention of night blindness and formation of visual purple in the eye
- Promotes bone growth, teeth development, reproduction
- Helps form and maintain healthy skin, hair, mucous membranes
- Builds body's resistance to respiratory and other infections (including measles in the Third World)

Possible Additional Benefits

- May help treat acne, impetigo, boils, carbuncles and open ulcers when applied externally
- May help control glaucoma
- Potential guard against effects of pollution and smog—beta-carotene acts as an antioxidant (see Glossary)
- May speed healing
- Possibly helps remove age spots
- May improve immunity
- May help heal skin lesions, cuts and wounds
- Possible treatment for hyperthyroidism

Who May Benefit from Additional Amounts?

- Anyone with inadequate caloric or nutritional dietary intake or increased nutritional requirements
- Those who abuse alcohol or other drugs
- People with a chronic wasting illness or prolonged fever
- Those under excess stress for long periods
- Anyone who has recently undergone surgery
- People with recent severe burns or injuries
- Malnourished children with impaired immunity

Deficiency Symptoms

- Night blindness
- Lack of tear secretion
- Changes in eyes—eventual blindness if deficiency is severe and untreated
- Susceptibility to infectious diseases, especially respiratory
- Dry, rough skin
- Weight loss
- Poor bone growth
- Weak tooth enamel
- Diarrhea
- Slow growth
- Acne
- Insomnia, fatigue

Usage Information

What this vitamin does:

- Essential for normal function of retina (combines with red pigment of retina—opsin—to form rhodopsin, which is necessary for sight in partial darkness)
- May act as cofactor (see Glossary) in enzyme systems
- Necessary for growth of bone, testicular function, ovarian function, embryonic development, regulation of growth, differentiation of tissues

Miscellaneous information:

- Many months of a vitamin-A-deficient diet are required before symptoms develop. The average person has a 2-year supply of vitamin A stored in the liver.
- Steroids are produced by the adrenal gland and are part of the natural response to stress and immune function. Failure to make these important hormones leaves the immune system in a less-than-ideal state.

Available as:

- Extended-release capsules or tablets: Swallow whole with a full glass of liquid. Don't chew or crush. Take with food or immediately after eating to decrease stomach irritation.
- Oral solution: Dilute in at least 1/2 glass of water or other liquid. Take with or 1 to 1-1/2 hours after meals unless otherwise directed by your doctor.
- Vitamin A is a constituent of many multivitamin/mineral preparations.
- Some forms are available by generic name.

Warnings and Precautions

Don't take if you are:

- Allergic to any preparation containing vitamin A.
- Planning a pregnancy or are pregnant and wish to take doses greater than the RDA.

Consult your doctor if you:

- Have cystic fibrosis
- Have diabetes
- Have intestinal disease with diarrhea
- Have kidney disease
- Have liver disease/liver enlargement
- Have overactive thyroid function
- Have disease of the pancreas
- Have viral hepatitis
- Have chronic alcoholism
- Are pregnant
- Are lactating

Over 55:

- Older people are more likely to be malnourished and need a supplement.
- Dosage must be taken carefully to avoid possible toxicity.

Pregnancy:

- Daily doses of retinol exceeding 5,000IU can produce growth retardation and urinary-tract malformations of the fetus.
- Don't take doses greater than RDA.

VITAMINS

→

Breastfeeding:
Don't take doses greater than RDA.

Effect on lab tests:
• Chronic vitamin-A toxicity—
  increased blood glucose, blood-urea
  nitrogen, serum calcium, serum
  cholesterol, serum triglycerides
• Poor results on dark-adaptation test
  (see Glossary)
• Poor results on electronystagmogram
  (see Glossary)
• Poor results on electroretinogram
  (see Glossary)

Storage:
• Store in cool, dry place away from
  direct light, but don't freeze.
• Store safely out of reach of children.
• Don't store in bathroom medicine
  cabinet. Heat and moisture may
  change the action of the vitamin.

Others:
• Children are more sensitive to
  vitamin A and are more likely to
  develop toxicity with dosages
  exceeding the RDA.
• Toxicity is slowly reversible on
  withdrawal of vitamin A but may
  persist for several weeks.

Overdose/Toxicity

Signs and symptoms:
Bleeding from gums or sore mouth;
bulging soft spot on head in babies;
sometimes hydrocephaly ("water on
brain"); confusion or unusual excitement; diarrhea; dizziness; double vision;
headache; irritability; dry skin; hair loss;
peeling skin on lips, palms and in
other areas; seizures; vomiting; enlarged
spleen and liver

Note: Toxicity symptoms usually
appear about 6 hours after ingestion of
overdoses of vitamin A. Symptoms may
also develop gradually if overdose is
mild and over a long period of time.
Overdose does not occur with beta-

carotene, but an excessive amount can
turn skin color to yellow-orange.

What to do:
For symptoms of overdose:
Discontinue vitamin and consult
doctor. Also see *Adverse Reactions or
Side Effects* section below.

For accidental overdose (such as
child taking entire bottle): Dial 911
(emergency), 0 for operator or call
your nearest Poison Control Center.

Adverse Reactions or Side Effects

Reaction or effect	What to do
Abdominal pain	Discontinue. Call doctor immediately.
Appetite loss	Discontinue. Call doctor when convenient.
Bone or joint pain	Discontinue. Call doctor immediately.
Discomfort, tiredness or weakness	Discontinue. Call doctor when convenient.
Drying or cracking of skin or lips	Discontinue. Call doctor immediately.
Fever	Discontinue. Call doctor immediately.
Hair loss	Discontinue. Call doctor immediately.
Headache	Discontinue. Call doctor when convenient.
Increase in frequency of urination	Discontinue. Call doctor when convenient.
Increased sensitivity of skin to sunlight	Discontinue. Call doctor when convenient.
Irritability	Discontinue. Call doctor when convenient.
Vomiting	Discontinue. Call doctor immediately.
Yellow-orange patches on soles of feet, palms of hands or skin around nose and lips	Consult doctor. Common with beta-carotene supplementation.

Interaction with Medicine, Minerals or Vitamins

Interacts with	Combined effect
Antacids	Decreases absorption of vitamin A and fat-soluble vitamins D, E and K.
Calcium supplements	Excessive vitamin A may decrease effect of calcium supplementation.
Cholestyramine, colestipol	Decreases absorption of vitamin A.
Mineral oil, neomycin	Decreases absorption of vitamin A.
Olestra-fat substitute	Decreases vitamin-A and beta-carotene absorption.
Oral contraceptives	Increases vitamin-A concentrations.
Retin-A	Used for acne treatment. Retin-A is a vitamin-A analog (see Glossary) and is contraindicated (see Glossary) during pregnancy and lactation.
Vitamin E	Normal amount facilitates absorption, storage in liver and utilization of vitamin A. Excessive dosage may deplete vitamin-A stores in liver. Long-term excess intake of beta-carotene can reduce vitamin-E levels.

Interaction with Other Substances

Tobacco decreases absorption. Smokers may need supplementary vitamin A.

Alcohol abuse interferes with the body's ability to transport and use vitamin A.

Lab Tests to Detect Deficiency

Many months of deficiency are required before lab studies reflect a deficiency.

- Plasma vitamin A and plasma carotene
- Dark-adaptation test
- Electronystagmogram
- Electroretinogram

VITAMINS

Ascorbic Acid (Vitamin C)

Basic Information

- Available from natural sources? Yes
- Available from synthetic sources? Yes
- Prescription required? No
- Water-soluble
- *Optimal Intake,* see pages 182–183

Natural Sources

Black currants
Broccoli
Brussels sprouts
Cabbage
Collards
Grapefruit
Green peppers
Guava
Kale
Lemons
Mangos

Orange juice
Oranges
Papayas
Peppers, sweet and hot
Potatoes
Rose hips
Spinach
Strawberries
Tangerines
Tomatoes
Watercress   ➜

Benefits

- Promotes healthy capillaries, gums, teeth
- Aids iron absorption
- Helps heal wounds, burns and broken bones
- Prevents and treats scurvy
- Part of treatment for anemia, especially for iron-deficiency anemia
- Part of treatment for urinary tract infections
- Helps form collagen in connective tissue
- Increases calcium absorption
- Contributes to hemoglobin and red-blood-cell production in bone marrow
- Blocks production of nitrosamines which are thought to be carcinogenic
- Aids adrenal gland function
- Reduces free-radical production

Possible Additional Benefits

- May prevent or reduce symptoms of the common cold and other infections
- May prevent some forms of cancer
- May reduce cholesterol
- Potential protection against heart disease
- Possible blood-clot prevention
- May prevent allergies
- May reduce symptoms of arthritis, skin ulcers, allergic reactions
- Possible relief of herpes infections of eyes and genitals
- May prevent periodontal disease
- May reduce toxic effect of alcohol and drugs
- May promote healing of bed sores
- May retard aging
- May improve male fertility

Who May Benefit from Additional Amounts?

- Anyone with inadequate caloric or nutritional dietary intake or increased nutritional requirements
- People more than 55 years old
- Those who abuse alcohol, tobacco or other drugs
- People with a chronic wasting illness, AIDS, acute illness with fever, hyperthyroidism, tuberculosis, cold exposure
- Those under excess stress for long periods
- Anyone who has recently undergone surgery
- Those with a portion of the gastrointestinal tract surgically removed
- People with recent severe burns or injuries
- Those receiving kidney dialysis
- Those who work in a toxic environment
- Anyone with the onset of infection symptoms

Deficiency Symptoms

- Scurvy: muscle weakness, swollen gums, loss of teeth, tiredness, depression, bleeding under skin, bleeding gums
- Easy bruising
- Swollen or painful joints
- Nosebleeds
- Anemia: weakness, tiredness, paleness
- Frequent infections
- Slow healing of wounds

Usage Information

What this vitamin does:
- Necessary for collagen formation and tissue repair

- Participates in oxidation-reduction reactions (see Glossary)
- Needed for metabolism of phenylalanine, tyrosine, folic acid, iron
- Aids utilization of carbohydrates, synthesis of fats and proteins, preservation of integrity of blood-vessel walls
- Strengthens blood vessels

Miscellaneous information:

Food preparation tips to conserve vitamin C:

- Eat food raw or minimally cooked.
- Shorten cooking time.
- Microwave or steam vegetables in very small amounts of water.
- Avoid leaving food at room temperature for prolonged period.
- Avoid overexposure of food to air and light.

Available as:

- Tablets: Swallow whole with a full glass of liquid. Don't chew or crush. Take with or 1 to 1-1/2 hours after meals unless otherwise directed by your doctor.
- Extended-release capsules or tablets: Swallow whole with a full glass of liquid. Don't chew or crush. Take with food or immediately after eating to decrease stomach irritation.
- Chewable tablets: Chew well before swallowing.
- Effervescent tablets: Allow to dissolve completely in liquid before swallowing.
- Oral solution: Dilute in at least 1/2 glass of water or other liquid. Take with or 1 to 1-1/2 hours after meals unless otherwise directed by your doctor.
- Injectable forms are administered by a doctor or nurse.
- Vitamin C is a constituent of many multivitamin/mineral preparations.

Warnings and Precautions

Don't take if you:
Are allergic to vitamin C.

Consult your doctor if you have:
- Gout
- Kidney stones
- Sickle-cell anemia
- Iron storage disease

Over 55:
- Needs may be greater because dietary intake tends to be lower.
- Side effects are more likely.

Pregnancy:
- Take prenatal vitamins with vitamin C because of the demands made by bone development, teeth and connective-tissue formation of fetus.
- If mother takes megadoses, newborn may develop deficiency symptoms after birth.
- Don't take doses greater than RDA.

Breastfeeding:
Continue taking prenatal vitamins to support rapid growth of child.

Effect on lab tests:
With megadoses (10 times recommended RDA):

- Blood in stool—possible false-negative test results with large doses
- LDH and SGOT (See Glossary)
- Glucose in urine—depends on method used
- Serum bilirubin—false low level
- Urinary pH—false low level

Storage:
- Store in a cool, dry place away from direct light, but don't freeze.
- Store safely out of reach of children.
- Don't store in bathroom medicine cabinet. Heat and moisture may change the action of the vitamin.

Others:
- Very high doses may cause kidney stones, although reported studies do not confirm this.

→

VITAMINS

- Recent studies show intake greater than 250mg/day in healthy persons is adequate to saturate the body's storage capacity.

 Overdose/Toxicity

Signs and symptoms:

Oral forms: flushed face, headache, increased urination, lower abdominal cramps, mild diarrhea, nausea, vomiting

Injectable forms: dizziness and faintness

What to do:

For symptoms of overdose: Discontinue vitamin and consult doctor. Also see *Adverse Reactions or Side Effects* section below.

For accidental overdose (such as child taking entire bottle): Dial 911 (emergency), 0 for operator or call your nearest Poison Control Center.

 Adverse Reactions or Side Effects

Reaction or effect	What to do
Anemia	Discontinue. Call doctor immediately.
Flushed face	Discontinue. Call doctor when convenient.
Headache	Discontinue. Call doctor when convenient.
Increased frequency of urination	Discontinue. Call doctor when convenient.
Lower abdominal cramps	Seek emergency treatment.
Mild diarrhea	Decrease dose. Call doctor when convenient.
Nausea or vomiting	Seek emergency treatment.
Rebound scurvy-like symptoms	Call doctor when convenient. If you decide to reduce dose, do so gradually to prevent deficiency symptoms.

 Interaction with Medicine, Minerals or Vitamins

Interacts with	Combined effect
Aminosalicylic acid (PAS for tuberculosis)	Increases chance of drug crystal formation in urine. Large doses of vitamin C must be taken to produce this effect.
Anticholinergics	Decreases anticholinergic effect.
Anticoagulants (oral)	Decreases anticoagulant effect.
Aspirin	Decreases vitamin-C effect.
Barbiturates	Decreases vitamin-C effect. Increases barbiturate effect.
Calcium	Assists in absorption of calcium.
Copper	Decreases absorption of copper. Large doses of vitamin C must be taken to produce this effect.
Iron supplements	Increases iron effect.
Quinidine	Decreases quinidine effect.
Salicylates	Decreases vitamin-C effect.
Sulfa drugs	Decreases vitamin-C effect. May cause kidney stones.
Tetracyclines	Decreases vitamin-C effect.

 Interaction with Other Substances

Tobacco decreases absorption. Smokers may require supplemental vitamin C.

Alcohol can be more rapidly broken down in body with large doses of vitamin C.

 Lab Tests to Detect Deficiency

- Vitamin-C levels in blood plasma
- Measurement of ascorbic-acid level in white blood cells (expensive and used mostly for experimental purposes)

Vitamin B-12

 ## Basic Information

Vitamin B-12 is also called *cyanocobalamin.*

- Available from natural sources? Yes
- Available from synthetic sources? Yes
- Prescription required? Yes, for high doses and injectable forms
- Water-soluble
- *Optimal Intake,* see pages 182–183

 ## Natural Sources

Beef	Liverwurst
Beef liver	Mackerel
Blue cheese	Milk
Clams	Oysters
Dairy products	Sardines
Eggs	Snapper
Flounder	Swiss cheese
Herring	

Note: Vitamin B-12 is not found in plant foods.

 ## Benefits

- Promotes normal growth and development
- Treats some types of nerve damage
- Treats pernicious anemia
- Treats and prevents vitamin B-12 deficiencies in people who have had a portion of the stomach or gastrointestinal tract surgically removed
- Prevents vitamin-B-12 deficiency in vegan vegetarians, persons with absorption diseases and elderly with achlorhydria
- Treats Alzheimer's disease

 ## Possible Additional Benefits

- Potential help to those with nervous disorders
- Possibly improves resistance to infection and disease
- May improve memory and the ability to learn
- May increase energy

 ## Who May Benefit from Additional Amounts?

- Strict vegetarians
- People with elevated homocysteine levels
- Anyone with inadequate caloric or nutritional dietary intake or increased nutritional requirements
- Those who abuse alcohol or other drugs
- People with a chronic wasting illness, AIDS or chronic fever
- Those under excess stress for long periods
- Anyone who has recently undergone surgery
- Those with a portion of the gastrointestinal tract surgically removed
- People with recent severe burns or injuries
- People with pancreas or bowel malignancy

 ## Deficiency Symptoms

Pernicious anemia, with the following symptoms:

- Fatigue, profound
- Weakness, especially in arms and legs
- Irreversible nerve damage

VITAMINS

- Sore tongue
- Nausea, appetite loss, weight loss
- Numbness and tingling in hands and feet
- Difficulty maintaining balance
- Pale lips, tongue and gums
- Shortness of breath
- Depression
- Confusion and dementia/disorientation
- Poor memory
- Bruising

Usage Information

What this vitamin does:
- Acts as coenzyme (see Glossary) for normal DNA synthesis (see Glossary)
- Promotes normal fat and carbohydrate metabolism and protein synthesis
- Promotes growth, cell development, blood-cell development, manufacture of nerve-cell covering, maintenance of normal nervous system function

Miscellaneous information:
There is a very low incidence of vitamin-B-12 toxicity, even with large amounts up to 1,000mcg/day.

Available as:
- Oral and injectable forms: Oral forms are used only as a diet supplement. Only people with portions of the gastrointestinal tract surgically removed or those with pernicious anemia require injections. Injectable forms are administered by a doctor or nurse.
- Tablets: Swallow whole with a full glass of liquid. Don't chew or crush. Take with or 1 to 1-1/2 hours after meals unless otherwise directed by your doctor.
- Extended-release capsules or tablets: Swallow whole with a full glass of liquid. Don't chew or crush. Take with food or immediately after eating to decrease stomach irritation.

- Vitamin B-12 is a constituent of many multivitamin/mineral preparations.

Warnings and Precautions

Don't take if you:
- Are allergic to B-12 given by injection (Allergy to injections produces itching, redness, swelling and, rarely, a blood-pressure drop with loss of consciousness.)
- Have Leber's disease

Consult your doctor if you have:
Anemia of unknown etiology (see Glossary). Folate supplementation can mask B-12 deficiency.

Over 55:
Absorption decreases in elderly with achlorhydria (decrease in hydrochloric acid in stomach).

Pregnancy:
- No problems are expected.
- Don't take doses greater than DRI.

Breastfeeding:
- No problems are expected.
- Don't take doses greater than DRI.

Effect on lab tests:
Tests for serum potassium may show precipitous drop (hypokalemia) within 48 hours after beginning treatment for anemia.

Storage:
- Store in a cool, dry place away from direct light, but don't freeze. Liquid forms should be refrigerated.
- Store safely out of reach of children.
- Don't store in bathroom medicine cabinet. Heat and moisture may change the action of the vitamin.

Others:
The injectable form is the only effective form to treat pernicious anemia or people with portions of the gastrointestinal tract surgically removed. These individuals do not absorb oral forms.

Overdose/Toxicity

Signs and symptoms:
If taken with large doses of vitamin C, vitamin B-12 may cause nosebleed, ear bleeding or dry mouth.

What to do:
For symptoms of overdose:
Discontinue vitamin and consult doctor. Also see *Adverse Reactions or Side Effects* section below.

For accidental overdose: (such as child taking entire bottle): Dial 911 (emergency), 0 for operator or call your nearest Poison Control Center.

Adverse Reactions or Side Effects

Reaction or effect	What to do
Diarrhea (rare)	Discontinue. Call doctor immediately.
Itching skin after injections (rare)	Seek emergency treatment.

Interaction with Medicine, Minerals or Vitamins

Interacts with	Combined effect
Aminosalicylates	Reduces absorption of vitamin B-12.
Antibiotics	May cause false low test results for vitamin B-12.
Chloramphenicol	May prevent therapeutic response when vitamin B-12 is used to treat anemia.
Cholestyramine	Reduces absorption of vitamin B-12.
Colchicine	Reduces absorption of vitamin B-12.
Epoetin	Reduces absorption of vitamin B-12.
Folic acid	Large doses mask deficiency of vitamin B-12.
Neomycin (oral forms)	Reduces absorption of vitamin B-12.
Potassium (extended-release forms)	Reduces absorption of vitamin B-12. May increase need for vitamin B-12.

Interaction with Other Substances

Tobacco decreases absorption. Smokers may require supplemental vitamin B-12.

Alcohol in excessive amounts for long periods may lead to vitamin B-12 deficiency.

Lab Tests to Detect Deficiency

• Serum vitamin B-12, a radioactive study usually performed with serum-folic-acid test, called the *Schilling test*
• Reticulocyte count

VITAMINS

Biotin (Vitamin H)

 Basic Information

- Available from natural sources? Yes
- Available from synthetic sources? No
- Prescription required? No
- Water-soluble

 Natural Sources

Almonds	Liver
Bananas	Mackerel
Brewer's yeast	Meats
Brown rice	Milk
Bulgur wheat	Mushrooms
Butter	Oat bran
Calf liver	Oatmeal
Cashew nuts	Peanut butter
Cheese	Peanuts
Chicken	Salmon
Clams	Soybeans
Eggs, cooked	Split peas
Green peas	Tuna
Lentils	Walnuts

 Benefits

- Aids formation of fatty acids
- Facilitates metabolism of amino acids and carbohydrates
- Promotes normal health of sweat glands, nerve tissue, bone marrow, male sex glands, blood cells, skin, hair
- Minimizes symptoms of zinc deficiency

 Possible Additional Benefits

- May alleviate muscle pain
- May alleviate depression

 Who May Benefit from Additional Amounts?

People who consume huge quantities of raw eggs, which contain a compound (avidin) that inhibits biotin. (Cooking eggs destroys this compound and eliminates the problem.)

 Deficiency Symptoms

Note: Deficiency is extremely rare.

Babies:
Dry scaling on scalp and face

Adults:
- Fatigue
- Depression
- Nausea
- Loss of appetite
- Loss of muscular reflexes
- Smooth, pale tongue
- Hair loss
- Increased blood-cholesterol levels
- Anemia
- Conjunctivitis
- Liver enlargement

 Usage Information

What this vitamin does:
Biotin is necessary for normal growth, development and health.

Miscellaneous information:
Intestinal bacteria produce all the biotin the body needs, so there is no substantial evidence that normal, healthy adults need dietary supplements of biotin.

Available as:
- Tablets or capsules: Swallow whole with a full glass of liquid. Don't chew or crush. Take with food or immediately after eating to decrease stomach irritation.
- Biotin is a constituent of many multivitamin/mineral preparations.

 ## Warnings and Precautions

Pregnancy:
No problems are expected.

Breastfeeding:
No problems are expected.

Storage:
- Store in a cool, dry place away from direct light, but don't freeze.
- Store safely out of reach of children.
- Don't store in bathroom medicine cabinet. Heat and moisture may change the action of the vitamin.

 ## Overdose/Toxicity

Signs and symptoms:
Supplements in amounts suggested by manufacturers on the label are nontoxic.

What to do:
For accidental overdose (such as child taking entire bottle): Dial 911 (emergency), 0 for operator or call your nearest Poison Control Center.

 ## Adverse Reactions or Side Effects

None are expected if taken within DRI dosage levels.

 ## Interaction with Medicine, Minerals or Vitamins

Interacts with	Combined effect
Long-term antibiotics (broad spectrum)	Destroys "friendly" bacteria in intestines that produce biotin. This can lead to significant biotin deficiency.
Sulfonamides	Destroys "friendly" bacteria in intestines that produce biotin. This can lead to significant biotin deficiency.

 ## Interaction with Other Substances

Tobacco decreases absorption. Smokers may require supplemental biotin.

Alcohol decreases absorption.

Foods: Eating large quantities of raw egg whites may cause biotin deficiency. Egg whites contain avidin, which prevents biotin from being absorbed into the body.

 ## Lab Tests to Detect Deficiency

None are available, except for experimental purposes.

VITAMINS

Choline

 Basic Information

- Choline is a precursor for acetylcholine.
- Available from natural sources? Yes
- Available from synthetic sources? Yes
- Prescription required? No
- *Optimal Intake*, see pages 182–183

 Natural Sources

Breast milk	Kale
Cabbage	Lentils
Calf liver	Oatmeal
Cauliflower	Peanuts
Egg yolk	Soybeans
Garbanzo beans	Soy lecithin
(chickpeas)	Wheat germ

 Benefits

- Maintains cell membrane integrity
- Choline is a component of lecithin, a structural component of cell walls
- Acetylcholine functions as a neurotransmitter

 Possible Additional Benefits

- May prevent some diseases of the nervous system, such as Alzheimer's disease, Huntington's disease and tardive dyskinesia (involuntary, abnormal facial movements including grimacing, sticking out tongue and sucking movements)
- May reduce symptoms of Alzheimer's disease
- May reduce liver damage caused by alcoholism and hepatitis
- May lower cholesterol level in human serum

 Who May Benefit From Additional Amounts?

No one

 Deficiency Symptoms

- Fatty deposition in liver
- Hemorrhagic kidney disease

 Usage Information

What this vitamin does:

Choline is involved in production of acetylcholine. Acetylcholine must be present in the body for proper function of the nervous system, including mood, behavior, orientation, personality traits, judgment.

Miscellaneous information:

- The major source for choline is lecithin. It is used as a thickener in several foods, including mayonnaise, margarine, ice cream.
- Humans can synthesize choline from ethanolamine and methyl groups derived from methionine.

Available as:

Capsules: Swallow whole with full glass of liquid. Don't chew or crush. Take with or 1 to 1-1/2 hours after meals unless otherwise directed by your doctor.

 Warnings and Precautions

Don't take if you:

Are healthy and eat a well-balanced diet.

Consult your doctor if you have:
Plans to use choline to treat Alzheimer's disease with lecithin/choline.

Over 55:
Don't take if you are healthy.

Pregnancy:
Don't take if you are healthy. Check with your doctor if you have any questions.

Breastfeeding:
Don't take if you are healthy. Check with your doctor if you have any questions.

Effect on lab tests:
May cause inaccurate results in choline/sphingomyelin test as part of examination of amniotic fluid.

Storage:
• Store in cool, dry place away from direct light, but don't freeze.
• Store safely out of reach of children.
• Don't store in bathroom medicine cabinet. Heat and moisture may change the action of the vitamin.

Others:
Don't take more than 1 gram per day.

Overdose/Toxicity

Signs and symptoms:
Nausea, vomiting, dizziness

What to do:
For symptoms of overdose:
Discontinue vitamin and consult doctor. Also see *Adverse Reactions or Side Effects* section below.

For accidental overdose (such as child taking entire bottle): Dial 911 (emergency), 0 for operator or call your nearest Poison Control Center.

Adverse Reactions or Side Effects

Reaction or effect	What to do
"Fishy" body odor	Discontinue. Call doctor when convenient.

Interaction with Medicine, Minerals or Vitamins

Interacts with	Combined effect
Methotrexate	Decreases choline absorption.
Nicotinic acid (nicotinamide, vitamin B-3)	Decreases choline effectiveness.
Phenobarbital	Decreases choline absorption.

Lab Tests to Detect Deficiency

Assessed by measuring serum-alanine amino-transferase levels

VITAMINS

Vitamin D

 Basic Information

Vitamin D is also called *cholecalciferol* or *sunshine vitamin.*

- Available from natural sources? Yes
- Available from synthetic sources? Yes
- Prescription required? No
- Fat-soluble
- *Optimal Intake,* see pages 182–183

 Natural Sources

Cod-liver oil
Egg substitutes
Halibut-liver oil
Herring
Mackerel
Salmon
Sardines
Sunlight
Tuna
Vitamin-D-fortified margarine
Vitamin-D-fortified milk

 Benefits

- Regulates growth, hardening and repair of bone by controlling absorption of calcium and phosphorus from small intestine
- Prevents rickets
- Treats hypocalcemia (low blood calcium) in those with kidney disease
- Treats post-operative muscle contractions
- Works with calcium to control bone formation
- Promotes normal growth and development of infants and children
- Promotes strong bones and teeth

 Possible Additional Benefits

- May reduce risk of breast or colon cancer
- Possible treatment for aging symptoms
- May treat vitamin-D malabsorption in those with cystic fibrosis

 Who May Benefit from Additional Amounts?

- Children who live in sunshine-deficient areas
- Anyone with inadequate caloric or nutritional dietary intake or increased nutritional requirements
- People more than 55 years old with limited sun exposure (for example, people who are institutionalized, use sunscreen or live in an area of limited sun exposure)
- Pregnant or breastfeeding women
- Those who abuse alcohol or other drugs
- People with a chronic wasting illness
- Those under excess stress for long periods
- Anyone who has recently undergone surgery
- Those with a portion of the gastrointestinal tract surgically removed
- People with recent severe burns or injuries
- Dark-skinned individuals
- Anyone with a liver impairment such as cirrhosis or obstructive jaundice (consult doctor)
- Breastfed babies
- Vegan vegetarians with limited sun exposure
- Those with cystic fibrosis

Deficiency Symptoms

- Rickets (a childhood deficiency disease): bent, bowed legs; malformations of joints or bones; late tooth development; weak muscles; listlessness
- Osteomalacia (adult rickets): pain in ribs, lower spine, pelvis and legs; muscle weakness and spasm; brittle, easily broken bones

Usage Information

What this vitamin does:

- Absorbs and uses calcium and phosphorus to make bone
- Essential for normal growth and development

Available as:

- Extended-release capsules or tablets: Swallow whole with a full glass of liquid. Don't chew or crush. Take with food or immediately after eating to decrease stomach irritation.
- Oral solution: Dilute in at least 1/2 glass of water or other liquid. Take with or 1 to 1-1/2 hours after meals unless otherwise directed by your doctor.
- Put liquid vitamin D directly into mouth or mix with cereal, fruit juice or food.
- Vitamin D is a constituent of many multivitamin/mineral preparations.
- Some forms are available by generic name.

Warnings and Precautions

Don't take if you:

Are allergic to vitamin D, ergocalciferol or any vitamin-D derivative.

Consult your doctor if you have:

- Any plans to become pregnant while taking vitamin D
- Epilepsy
- Heart or blood-vessel disease
- Kidney, liver or pancreatic disease
- Chronic diarrhea
- Intestinal problems
- Sarcoidosis

Over 55:

Adverse reactions and side effects are more likely. Supplements may be necessary.

Pregnancy:

- Taking too much during pregnancy may cause abnormalities in the fetus. Consult doctor before taking a supplement to ensure correct dosage.
- Don't take doses greater than DRI.

Breastfeeding:

- It is important to receive the correct amount so enough vitamin D is available for normal growth and development of baby. Consult doctor about supplements.
- Don't take doses greater than DRI.

Effect on lab tests:

- May decrease serum alkaline phosphatase
- May increase levels of calcium, cholesterol and phosphate in test results
- May increase level of magnesium in test results
- May increase amounts of calcium and phosphorus in urine

Storage:

- Store in a cool, dry place away from direct light, but don't freeze. Avoid overexposure to air.
- Store safely out of reach of children.
- Don't store in bathroom medicine cabinet. Heat and moisture may change the action of the vitamin.

Others:

- Absence of sunlight prevents natural formation of vitamin D by skin. ➔

VITAMINS

Sunshine provides sufficient amounts of vitamin D for people who live in sunny climates. Those who live in northern areas with fewer days of sunshine and extended periods of cloud cover and darkness must depend on dietary sources for vitamin D.
• Avoid doses greater than DRI.

Overdose/Toxicity

Signs and symptoms:
High blood pressure, irregular heartbeat, nausea, weight loss, seizures, abdominal pain, appetite loss, mental- and physical-growth retardation, premature hardening of arteries, kidney damage

What to do:
For symptoms of overdose:
Discontinue vitamin and consult doctor. Also see *Adverse Reactions or Side Effects* section below.

For accidental overdose (such as child taking entire bottle): Dial 911 (emergency), 0 for operator or call your nearest Poison Control Center.

For toxic symptoms: Discontinue vitamin and seek immediate medical help. Hospitalization may be necessary.

Adverse Reactions or Side Effects

Reaction or effect	What to do
Appetite loss	Discontinue. Call doctor when convenient.
Constipation	Discontinue. Call doctor when convenient.
Diarrhea	Discontinue. Call doctor immediately.
Dry mouth	Discontinue. Call doctor when convenient.
Headache	Discontinue. Call doctor immediately.
Increased thirst	Discontinue. Call doctor when convenient.
Mental confusion	Discontinue. Call doctor immediately.
Metallic taste	Discontinue. Call doctor when convenient.
Nausea or vomiting	Discontinue. Call doctor immediately.
Unusual tiredness	Discontinue. Call doctor when convenient.

Interaction with Medicine, Minerals or Vitamins

Interacts with	Combined effect
Antacids with aluminum	Decreases absorption of vitamin D and fat-soluble vitamins A, E and K.
Antacids with magnesium	May cause too much magnesium in blood, especially in people with kidney failure.
Anticonvulsants	May reduce effect of vitamin D from natural sources and require supplements to prevent loss of strength in bones.
Barbiturates	May reduce effect of vitamin D from natural sources and require supplements to prevent loss of strength in bones.
Calcitonin	Reduces effect of calcitonin when treating hypercalcemia.
Calcium (high doses)	Increases risk of hypercalcemia.
Cholestyramine	Impairs absorption of vitamin D. May need supplements.
Colestipol	Impairs absorption of vitamin D. May need supplements.
Cortisone	Decreases absorption of vitamin D.
Digitalis preparations	Increases risk of heartbeat irregularities.

Diuretics, thiazide	Increases risk of hypercalcemia.
Hydantoin	May reduce effect of vitamin D from natural sources and require supplements to prevent loss of strength in bones.
Mineral oil	Increases absorption of vitamin D. May need supplements.
Phosphorus-containing medicines	Increases risk of too much phosphorus in blood.
Primidone	May reduce effect of vitamin D from natural sources and require supplements to prevent loss of strength in bones.
Vitamin-D derivatives, such as calciferol, calcitrol, dihydrotachysterol, ergocalciferol	Additive effects may increase potential for toxicity.

Interaction with Other Substances

Alcohol abuse depletes liver stores of vitamin D.

Olestra fat substitute can decrease absorption of vitamin D.

Lab Tests to Detect Deficiency

- Reduced levels of vitamin-D forms in blood
- Decreased serum phosphate and calcium, increased alkaline phosphatase, urinary hydroxyproline, parathyroid hormone (PTH) levels
- Bone X-ray

VITAMINS

Vitamin E

Basic Information

Vitamin E is also called *alpha-tocopherol.*

D alpha-tocopherol is the most absorbable.

- Available from natural sources? Yes
- Available from synthetic sources? Yes
- Prescription required? No, except for injectable forms
- Fat-soluble
- *Optimal Intake,* see pages 182–183

Natural Sources

Almonds	Fortified cereals
Asparagus	Hazelnuts (filberts)
Avocados	Peanuts/oil
Brazil nuts	Safflower nuts/oil
Broccoli	Soybean oil
Canola oil	Spinach
Corn	Sunflower seeds
Corn oil/margarine	Walnuts
Cottonseed oil	Wheat germ
	Wheat-germ oil

Benefits

- Promotes normal growth and development

→

- Treats and prevents vitamin-E deficiency in premature or low-birthweight infants
- Acts as anti-blood-clotting agent
- Promotes normal red-blood-cell formation
- Promotes vitamin-C recycling
- Reduces risk of fatal first myocardial infarction in men
- Protects against prostate cancer
- Improves immunity—especially in vitamin-E deficient people
- Antioxidant (see Glossary) for cancer, heart disease, tissue, free radicals in the body

Possible Additional Benefits

- May reduce symptoms of fibrocystic disease of breast
- May reduce circulatory problems of lower extremities
- Possible coronary artery heart disease prevention
- Potentially enhances sexual performance
- May improve muscle strength and stamina
- May promote healing of burns and wounds
- May retard aging
- Possible relief from menopausal symptoms
- Potential treatment for bee stings, diaper rash
- May decrease scar formation
- May improve athletic performance
- Possible acne treatment
- May prevent eye and lung problems in low-birthweight or premature infants
- May treat skin disorders associated with lupus
- Possibly reduces blood glucose levels in some diabetics
- May protect against macular degeneration, cataracts

Who May Benefit from Additional Amounts?

- Anyone with inadequate caloric or nutritional dietary intake or increased nutritional requirements
- People more than 55 years old
- Those who abuse alcohol or other drugs
- People who have a chronic wasting illness
- Those under excess stress for long periods
- Anyone who has recently undergone surgery
- Those with liver, gallbladder or pancreatic disease
- People with recent severe burns or injuries
- People with hyperthyroidism
- Anyone at risk for myocardial infarction
- People with cystic fibrosis
- People with celiac disease

Deficiency Symptoms

Premature infants and children:
- Irritability
- Edema
- Hemolytic anemia

Adults:
- Lethargy
- Apathy
- Inability to concentrate
- Nerve dysfunction

Usage Information

What this vitamin does:
- Prevents a chemical reaction called *oxidation* (see Glossary)—excessive oxidation can sometimes cause harmful effects
- Acts as a cofactor (see Glossary) in several enzyme systems

Miscellaneous information:

- Vitamin E is a constituent of many skin ointments, salves and creams. Claims for beneficial effects have not been confirmed, but topical application probably does not cause harm.
- Several weeks of treatment may be necessary before symptoms caused by a deficiency will improve.
- Freezing may destroy vitamin E.
- Extreme heat causes vitamin E to break down. Avoid deep-fat frying foods that are natural sources of vitamin E.
- Vitamin E functions as an antioxidant (see Glossary), prevents enzyme action of peroxidase on unsaturated bonds of cell membranes and protects red blood cells from disintegrating.

Available as:

- Tablets or capsules: Swallow whole with a full glass of liquid. Don't chew or crush. Take with food or immediately after eating to decrease stomach irritation.
- Drops: Dilute dose in beverage before swallowing, or squirt directly into mouth.
- Vitamin E is a constituent of many multivitamin/mineral preparations.

Warnings and Precautions

Don't take if you are:

- Allergic to vitamin E
- Taking coumadin

Consult your doctor if you have:

- Iron-deficiency anemia
- Bleeding or clotting problems
- Cystic fibrosis
- Intestinal problems
- Liver disease
- Overactive thyroid
- Low-birthweight baby (supplementation appears to increase immune function)

Pregnancy:

- No problems are expected, except with doses greater than RDA.
- Low-birthweight babies are at risk for vitamin-E deficiency.

Breastfeeding:

No problems are expected.

Effect on lab tests:

Serum cholesterol and serum triglycerides may register high if you take large doses of vitamin E.

Storage:

- Store in a cool, dry place away from direct light, but don't freeze.
- Store safely out of reach of children.
- Don't store in bathroom medicine cabinet. Heat and moisture may change the action of the vitamin.

Others:

Beware of doses greater than RDA.

Overdose/Toxicity

Signs and symptoms:

High doses deplete vitamin-A stores in body. Very high doses (over 1,000IU/day) may cause nausea; flatulence; headache; fainting; diarrhea; tendency to bleed; altered immunity; impaired sex functions; increased risk of blood clots; altered metabolism of thyroid, pituitary and adrenal hormones.

What to do:

For accidental overdose (such as a child taking entire bottle): Dial 911 (emergency), 0 for operator or call your nearest Poison Control Center.

For symptoms of toxicity:

Discontinue vitamin and consult doctor. Also see *Adverse Reactions or Side Effects* section below.

VITAMINS

➜

Adverse Reactions or Side Effects

Reaction or effect	What to do
Abdominal pain	Discontinue. Call doctor immediately.
Breast enlargement	Discontinue. Call doctor when convenient.
Diarrhea	Discontinue. Call doctor immediately.
Dizziness	Discontinue. Call doctor when convenient.
Flu-like symptoms	Discontinue. Call doctor immediately.
Headache	Discontinue. Call doctor when convenient.
Nausea	Discontinue. Call doctor immediately.
Tiredness or weakness	Discontinue. Call doctor when convenient.
Vision blurred	Discontinue. Call doctor immediately.

Interaction with Medicine, Minerals or Vitamins

Interacts with	Combined effect
Antacids	Decreases vitamin-E absorption.
Anticoagulants, coumadin- or indandione-type	May increase spontaneous or hidden bleeding.
Aspirin (long-term use)	May reduce blood clotting to greater extent than desired to decrease cardiac disease.
Cholestyramine	May decrease absorption of vitamin E.
Colestipol	May decrease absorption of vitamin E.
Iron supplements	Decreases effect of iron with iron-deficiency anemia. Decreases vitamin-E effect in healthy people.
Mineral oil	May decrease absorption of vitamin E.
Sucralfate	May decrease absorption of vitamin E.
Vitamin A	Facilitates absorption, storage and utilization of vitamin A. Reduces potential toxicity of vitamin A. Excessive doses of vitamin E cause vitamin-A depletion.

Interaction with Other Substances

Tobacco decreases absorption. Smokers may require supplemental vitamin E.

Alcohol abuse depletes vitamin-E stores in tissue.

Olestra fat substitute reduces absorption of vitamin E.

Lab Tests to Detect Deficiency

- Blood tocopherol level
- Excess creatine in urine to indicate muscle breakdown
- Red-blood-cell fragility test

Folic Acid (Vitamin B-9, Folate)

Basic Information

Folic acid is also called *pteroylglutamic acid* and *folacin*.

Folate comes from dietary sources.

Folic acid comes from supplements.

- Available from natural sources? Yes
- Available from synthetic sources? Yes
- Prescription required? No
- Water-soluble
- *Optimal Intake,* see pages 182–183

Natural Sources

Asparagus	Citrus fruits/juices
Avocados	Endive
Bananas	Fortified grain products
Beans	Garbanzo beans
Beets	(chickpeas)
Brewer's yeast	Green, leafy
Brussels sprouts	vegetables
Cabbage	Lentils
Calf liver	Sprouts
Cantaloupe	Wheat germ

Benefits

- Promotes normal red-blood-cell formation
- Maintains nervous system, intestinal tract, sex organs, white blood cells, normal patterns of growth
- Regulates embryonic and fetal development of nerve cells and prevents neural-tube defects
- Promotes normal growth and development
- Treats anemias due to folic-acid deficiency occurring from alcoholism, liver disease, hemolytic anemia, sprue, pregnancy, breastfeeding, oral-contraceptive use
- Aids metabolism of amino acids and protein synthesis (RNA, DNA)

Possible Additional Benefits

B-9 may reduce cervical dysplasia.

Who May Benefit from Additional Amounts?

- Anyone with inadequate caloric or nutritional dietary intake or increased nutritional requirements
- People more than 55 years old with inadequate dietary intake
- Pregnant or breastfeeding women
- Women who use oral contraceptives
- Those who abuse alcohol or other drugs
- People with a chronic wasting illness, AIDS/HIV
- Those under excess stress for long periods
- Those with a portion of the gastrointestinal tract surgically removed
- People with recent severe burns or injuries
- Women capable of becoming pregnant

Deficiency Symptoms

- Megaloblastic anemia, in which red blood cells are large and uneven in size

VITAMINS

→

- Irritability
- Weakness
- Lack of energy
- Loss of appetite
- Paleness
- Sore, red tongue
- Mild mental symptoms, such as forgetfulness and confusion
- Diarrhea

Usage Information

What this vitamin does:
- Acts as coenzyme (see Glossary) for normal DNA synthesis
- Functions as part of coenzyme in amino acid and nucleoprotein synthesis
- Promotes normal red-blood-cell formation

Miscellaneous information:
- Cooking vegetables causes loss of some folate content.
- In January 1998 the USDA began a fortification program to increase folate content of grain- and flour-containing products.

Available as:
- Tablets: Swallow whole with a full glass of liquid. Don't chew or crush. Take with or 1 to 1-1/2 hours after meals unless otherwise directed by your doctor.

Warnings and Precautions

Don't take if you:
- Have pernicious anemia (Folic acid will make the blood appear normal, but neurological problems may progress and be irreversible.)
- Take anticonvulsant medication

Consult your doctor if you:
- Have anemia
- Are taking methotrexate

Pregnancy:
- No problems are expected.
- Don't take doses greater than DRI.

Breastfeeding:
- No problems are expected.
- Don't take doses greater than DRI.

Effect on lab tests:
May cause false low results in tests for vitamin B-12.

Storage:
- Store in a cool, dry place away from direct light, but don't freeze.
- Store safely out of reach of children.
- Don't store in bathroom medicine cabinet. Heat and moisture may change the action of the vitamin.

Others:
Renal dialysis reduces blood folate. Patients on dialysis should increase intake to more than 400mg/day.

Overdose/Toxicity

Signs and symptoms:
Prolonged use of high doses can produce damaging folacin crystals in the kidney. Doses over 1,500mcg/day can cause appetite loss, nausea, flatulence, abdominal distension and may obscure existence of pernicious anemia.

What to do:

For symptoms of overdose:
Discontinue vitamin and consult doctor. Also see *Adverse Reactions or Side Effects* section below.

For accidental overdose (such as child taking entire bottle): Dial 911 (emergency), 0 for operator or call your nearest Poison Control Center.

Adverse Reactions or Side Effects

Reaction or effect	What to do
Bright-yellow urine (always)	Nothing.
Diarrhea	Discontinue. Call doctor.
Fever	Discontinue. Call doctor immediately.
Shortness of breath due to anemia	Discontinue. Call doctor immediately.
Skin rash	Discontinue. Call doctor when convenient.

Interaction with Medicine, Minerals or Vitamins

Interacts with	Combined effect
Analgesics	Decreases effect of folic acid.
Antacids containing aluminum or magnesium	Prolonged use may decrease absorption of folic acid. Take folic acid two hours before taking an antacid.
Antibiotics	May cause false low results in tests for serum folic acid.
Anticonvulsants	Decreases effect of folic acid and anticonvulsant.
Chloramphenicol	Produces folic-acid deficiency.
Cortisone drugs	Decreases effect of folic acid.
Epoetin	Decreases effect of folic acid.
Methotrexate	Decreases effect of folic acid. Methotrexate is a folate antagonist (see Glossary).
Oral contraceptives	Those who take oral contraceptives may require additional folic acid or dietary folate.
Phenytoin	Decreases phenytoin effect. Patients taking phenytoin should avoid taking folic acid.
Pyrimethamine	Decreases effect of folic acid and interferes with effectiveness of pyrimethamine. Avoid this combination.
Quinine	Decreases effect of folic acid.
Sulfasalazine and other sulfa drugs	Decreases effect of folic acid.
Triamterene	Decreases effect of folic acid.
Trimethoprim	Decreases effect of folic acid.

Interaction with Other Substances

Tobacco decreases absorption. Smokers may require supplemental folic acid.

Alcohol abuse makes deficiency more likely. Alcoholism is the principal cause of folic-acid deficiency.

Lab Tests to Detect Deficiency

- Serum folate
- Blood cells showing macrocytic anemia coupled with normal levels of B-12 in blood
- Red-blood-cell (RBC) folate

VITAMINS

Niacin (Vitamin B-3)

Basic Information

- Available from natural sources? Yes
- Available from synthetic sources? Yes
- Prescription required? Yes, for high doses used for cholesterol reduction
- Water-soluble
- *Optimal Intake,* see pages 182–183

Natural Sources

Beef liver	Peanuts
Brewer's yeast	Pork/ham
Chicken,	Potatoes
white meat	Salmon
Dried beans/peas	Soybeans
Fortified cereals	Swordfish
Halibut	Tuna
Peanut butter	Turkey

Benefits

- Treats pellagra (see Glossary)
- Corrects niacin deficiency
- Reduces cholesterol and triglycerides in blood
- Dilates blood vessels if taken in doses larger than 75mg (consult doctor)
- Treats vertigo (dizziness) and ringing in ears

Possible Additional Benefits

- May reduce risk of heart attacks
- May reduce depression
- May reduce migraine headaches
- Potentially improves poor digestion

Who May Benefit from Additional Amounts?

- Anyone with inadequate caloric or nutritional dietary intake or increased nutritional requirements
- People more than 55 years old with poor dietary intake
- Pregnant or breastfeeding women
- Those who abuse alcohol or other drugs
- People with a chronic wasting illness, including malignancies, pancreatic insufficiency, cirrhosis of the liver, sprue
- People with recent severe burns or injuries
- Infants born with errors of metabolism (congenital disorders due to chromosome abnormalities)

Deficiency Symptoms

Early symptoms:

- Delirium
- General fatigue/lethargy
- Loss of appetite
- Headaches
- Swollen, red tongue
- Skin lesions, including rashes, dry scaly skin, wrinkles, coarse skin texture
- Indigestion
- Dermatitis/dark pigmentation
- Diarrhea
- Irritability
- Dizziness

Late symptoms of severe deficiency, called *pellagra:*

- Dementia
- Death

Usage Information

What this vitamin does:

• Aids in release of energy from foods
• Helps synthesize DNA
• Becomes component of two coenzymes (see Glossary), NAD and NADP, which are both necessary for utilization of fats, tissue respiration and production of sugars

Miscellaneous information:

• The body manufactures niacin from tryptophan, an amino acid.
• Vitamin B-6 is needed to convert tryptophan to niacin.
• Long-term, high-dose leucine supplementation can cause tryptophan and niacin deficiency.

Available as:

• Tablets or capsules: Swallow whole with a full glass of liquid. Don't chew or crush. Take with or 1 to 1-1/2 hours after meals unless otherwise directed by your doctor.
• Extended-release capsules or tablets: Swallow whole with a full glass of liquid. Don't chew or crush. Take with food or immediately after eating to decrease stomach irritation.
• Oral solution: Dilute in at least 1/2 glass of water or other liquid. Take with or 1 to 1-1/2 hours after meals unless otherwise directed by your doctor.
• Injectable forms are administered by a doctor or nurse.
• Niacin is a constituent of most multivitamin/mineral preparations.
• Some forms are available by generic name.

 ## Warnings and Precautions

Don't take if you:

• Are allergic to niacin or any niacin-containing vitamin mixtures
• Have impaired liver function
• Have an active peptic ulcer

Consult your doctor if you have:

• Diabetes
• Gout
• Gallbladder or liver disease
• Arterial bleeding
• Glaucoma

Over 55:

Response to niacin cannot be predicted. Dose must be individualized.

Pregnancy:

Risk to fetus with high doses outweighs benefits. Do not use.

Breastfeeding:

• Studies are inconclusive. Consult doctor about supplements.
• Don't take doses greater than DRI.

Effect on lab tests:

• Urinary catecholamine concentration may falsely elevate results.
• Urine glucose (using Benedict's reagent) may produce false-positive reactions.
• Niacin can elevate blood sugar and falsely increase growth-hormone level in blood.
• Large daily doses may elevate blood uric acid.

Storage:

• Store in a cool, dry place away from direct light, but don't freeze.
• Store safely out of reach of children.
• Don't store in bathroom medicine cabinet. Heat and moisture may change the action of the vitamin.

VITAMINS

Others:
High dosages over long periods may cause liver damage or aggravate a stomach ulcer.

Overdose/Toxicity

Signs and symptoms:
Body flush, nausea, diarrhea, weakness, lightheadedness, headache, fainting, high blood sugar, high uric acid, heart-rhythm disturbances, jaundice.

What to do:
For symptoms of overdose:
Discontinue vitamin and consult doctor. Also see *Adverse Reactions or Side Effects* section below.

For accidental overdose (such as child taking entire bottle): Dial 911 (emergency), 0 for operator or call your nearest Poison Control Center.

Adverse Reactions or Side Effects

Reaction or effect	What to do
Abdominal pain	Discontinue. Call doctor immediately.
Darkening of urine	Nothing.
Diarrhea	Discontinue. Call doctor when convenient.
Faintness	Discontinue. Call doctor immediately.
Headache	Discontinue. Call doctor when convenient.
"Hot" feeling, with skin flushed in blush zone (always)	Nothing.
Jaundice (yellow skin and eyes)	Discontinue. Call doctor immediately.
Nausea or vomiting	Discontinue. Call doctor immediately.
Skin dryness	Discontinue. Call doctor when convenient.

Interaction with Medicine, Minerals or Vitamins

Interacts with	Combined effect
Antidiabetics	Decreases antidiabetic effect.
Beta-adrenergic blockers	Lowers blood pressure to extremely low level.
Chenodiol	Decreases chenodiol effect.
Guanethidine	Increases guanethidine effect.
HMG-CoA reductase inhibitors	Increases risk of rhabdomyolysis and renal failure.
Isoniazid	Decreases niacin effect.
Mecamylamine	Lowers blood pressure to extremely low level.
Pargyline	Lowers blood pressure to extremely low level.
Ursodiol	Decreases ursodiol effect.

Interaction with Other Substances

Tobacco decreases absorption. Smokers may require supplemental niacin.

Alcohol may cause extremely low blood pressure. Use caution.

Lab Tests to Detect Deficiency

- Urinary N-1 methylnicotinamide
- Urinary 2-pyridone/N-1 methylnicotinamide—test results not always conclusive

Pantothenic Acid (Vitamin B-5)

Basic Information

- Available from natural sources? Yes
- Available from synthetic sources? Yes
- Prescription required? No
- Water-soluble
- *Optimal Intake,* see pages 182–183

Natural Sources

Avocados	Meats, all kinds
Bananas	Milk
Blue cheese	Oranges
Broccoli	Peanut butter
Chicken	Peanuts
Collard greens	Peas
Eggs	Soybeans
Lentils	Sunflower seeds
Liver	Wheat germ
Lobster	Whole-grain products

Benefits

- Promotes normal growth and development
- Aids release of energy from foods
- Helps synthesize numerous body materials

Possible Additional Benefits

- May stimulate wound healing in animals
- May alleviate stress
- May reduce fatigue

Who May Benefit from Additional Amounts?

- Anyone with inadequate caloric or nutritional dietary intake or increased nutritional requirements
- People more than 55 years old with vitamin-B deficiencies
- Pregnant or breastfeeding women
- Those who abuse alcohol or other drugs
- People with a chronic wasting illness, including sprue, celiac disease, regional enteritis
- Those under excess stress for long periods
- Anyone who has recently undergone surgery
- Athletes and workers who participate in vigorous physical activities

Deficiency Symptoms

No proven symptoms exist for pantothenic acid alone. However, lack of one B vitamin usually means lack of other B nutrients. Pantothenic acid is usually given with other B vitamins if there are symptoms of any vitamin-B deficiency, including excessive fatigue, sleep disturbances, loss of appetite, nausea or dermatitis.

Usage Information

What this vitamin does:

Vitamin B-5 is converted to a coenzyme (see Glossary) in energy metabolism of carbohydrates, protein and fat.

VITAMINS

➜

Available as:
- Tablets: Swallow whole with a full glass of liquid. Don't chew or crush. Take with or 1 to 1-1/2 hours after meals unless otherwise directed by your doctor.
- Vitamin B-5 is a constituent of many multivitamin/mineral preparations and B-complex vitamins.

 # Warnings and Precautions

Don't take if you are:
- Allergic to pantothenic acid
- Taking levodopa for Parkinson's disease

Consult your doctor if you have:
Hemophilia.

Pregnancy:
Don't exceed recommended dose.

Breastfeeding:
Don't exceed recommended dose.

Storage:
- Store in a cool, dry place away from direct light, but don't freeze.
- Store safely out of reach of children.
- Don't store in bathroom medicine cabinet. Heat and moisture may change the action of the vitamin.

Others:
Avoid doses greater than five times the DRI.

 # Overdose/Toxicity

What to do:
For symptoms of overdose:
Discontinue vitamin and consult doctor. Also see *Adverse Reactions or Side Effects* section below.

For accidental overdose (such as child taking entire bottle): Dial 911 (emergency), 0 for operator or call your nearest Poison Control Center.

 # Adverse Reactions or Side Effects

Reaction or effect	What to do
Diarrhea	Discontinue or reduce close to DRI levels.

 # Interaction with Medicine, Minerals or Vitamins

Interacts with	Combined effect
Levodopa	Small amounts of pantothenic acid nullify levodopa's effect. Carbidopa-levodopa combination is not affected by this interaction.

 # Interaction with Other Substances

Tobacco decreases absorption. Smokers may require supplemental pantothenic acid.

 # Lab Tests to Detect Deficiency

Methods are limited and expensive. Tests are used only for research at present. Methods are available to measure blood levels and levels in 24-hour urine collections.

Phytonadione (Vitamin K)

Basic Information

Phytonadione and *menadiol* are forms of vitamin K.

- Available from natural sources? Yes
- Available from synthetic sources? Yes
- Prescription required? Yes
- Fat-soluble
- *Optimal Intake,* see pages 182–183

Natural Sources

Alfalfa	Green, leafy lettuce
Asparagus	Liver
Broccoli	Seaweed
Brussels sprouts	Spinach
Cabbage	Turnip greens
Cheddar cheese	

Benefits

- Promotes normal growth and development
- Prevents hemorrhagic disease of the newborn
- Treats bleeding disorders due to vitamin-K deficiency
- Regulates normal blood clotting
- Promotes bone health

Possible Additional Benefits

None are known.

Who May Benefit from Additional Amounts?

- Those with a portion of the gastrointestinal tract surgically removed
- All newborns
- Anyone taking long-term antibiotics that may destroy normal "friendly" bacteria in the intestinal tract
- People who do not have enough bile to absorb fats (replacement must be given by injection or in water-soluble form)
- Infants who are breastfed or fed with milk-substitute formula
- People on mineral oil (for constipation)

Deficiency Symptoms

Infants:

- Failure to grow and develop normally
- Hemorrhagic disease of the newborn characterized by vomiting blood and bleeding from intestine, umbilical cord, circumcision site (symptoms begin 2 or 3 days after birth)

Adults:

Abnormal blood clotting that can lead to

- nosebleeds
- blood in urine
- stomach bleeding
- bleeding from capillaries or skin, causing spontaneous black-and-blue marks
- prolonged clotting time (a laboratory test)

VITAMINS

→

Usage Information

What this vitamin does:

Promotes production of active prothrombin (factor II), proconvertin (factor VII) and other factors necessary for normal blood clotting.

Miscellaneous information:

- Very little vitamin K is lost from processing or cooking foods.
- When a severe bleeding disorder exists due to a vitamin-K deficiency, fresh whole blood may be needed during severe bleeding episodes.

Available as:

- Tablets: Swallow whole with a full glass of liquid. Don't chew or crush. Take with or 1 to 1-1/2 hours after meals unless otherwise directed by your doctor.
- Injectable forms are administered by a doctor or nurse.
- Water-soluble tablets and liquids are also available.

Note: Vitamin K is not usually included in most multivitamin/mineral preparations.

 Warnings and Precautions

Don't take if you:

- Are allergic to vitamin K
- Have a G6PD deficiency (see Glossary)
- Have liver disease

Consult your doctor if you have:

- Cystic fibrosis
- Prolonged diarrhea
- Prolonged intestinal problems
- Taken any other medicines
- Plans for surgery (including dental surgery) in the near future

Over 55:

- No problems are expected.
- Don't take doses greater than RDA.

Pregnancy:

- No studies are available in humans. Avoid if possible.
- Don't take doses greater than RDA.

Breastfeeding:

Don't take doses greater than RDA.

Effect on lab tests:

Changes prothrombin times.

Storage:

- Store in a cool, dry place away from direct light, but don't freeze.
- Store safely out of reach of children.
- Don't store in bathroom medicine cabinet. Heat and moisture may change the action of the vitamin.

Others:

- Avoid overdosage. Vitamin K is a fat-soluble vitamin. Excess intake can lead to impaired liver function.
- Tell any dentist or doctor who plans surgery that you take vitamin K.

 Overdose/Toxicity

Signs and symptoms:

Brain damage in infants and impaired liver function in infants and adults who take large doses.

What to do:

For symptoms of overdose:

Discontinue vitamin and consult doctor. Also see *Adverse Reactions or Side Effects* section below.

For accidental overdose (such as child taking entire bottle): Dial 911 (emergency), 0 for operator or call your nearest Poison Control Center.

Adverse Reactions or Side Effects

Reaction or effect	What to do
Hemolytic anemia in infants	Seek emergency treatment.
Hyperbilirubinemia (too much bilirubin in the blood) in newborns or infants given too much vitamin K, marked by jaundice (yellow skin and eyes)	Seek emergency treatment.

Allergic reactions, including:

Face flushing	Discontinue. Call doctor immediately.
Gastrointestinal upset	Discontinue. Call doctor immediately.
Rash	Discontinue. Call doctor immediately.
Redness, pain or swelling at injection site	Discontinue. Call doctor immediately.
Skin itching	Seek emergency treatment.

Interaction with Medicine, Minerals or Vitamins

Interacts with	Combined effect
Antacids (long-term use)	Large amounts may interfere with vitamin-K effect.
Antibiotics, broad spectrum (long-term use)	Causes vitamin-K deficiency.
Anticoagulants (oral)	Decreases anticoagulant effect.
Cholestyramine	Decreases vitamin-K absorption.
Colestipol	Decreases vitamin-K absorption.
Coumarin (isolated from sweet clover)	Decreases vitamin-K effect.
Dactinomycin	May decrease vitamin-K effect.
Hemolytics	Increases potential for toxic side effects.
Mineral oil (long-term use)	Causes vitamin-K deficiency.
Primaquine	Increases potential for toxic side effects.
Quinidine	Causes vitamin-K deficiency.
Salicylates	Increases need for vitamin K when administered over long time.
Sucralfate	Decreases vitamin-K effect.
Sulfa drugs	Causes vitamin-K deficiency.

Lab Tests to Detect Deficiency

- Prothrombin time
- Serum prothrombin
- Serum vitamin K

VITAMINS

Pyridoxine (Vitamin B-6)

 ## Basic Information

Pyridoxine is also called *pyridoxal phosphate.*

- Available from natural sources? Yes
- Available from synthetic sources? Yes
- Prescription required? No
- Water-soluble
- *Optimal Intake,* see pages 182–183

 ## Natural Sources

Avocados
Bananas
Beef liver
Chicken
Fortified cereals
Ground beef
Ham
Hazelnuts (filberts)

Lentils
Potatoes
Salmon
Shrimp
Soybeans
Sunflower seeds
Tuna
Wheat germ

 ## Benefits

- Participates actively in many chemical reactions of proteins and amino acids
- Helps normal function of brain
- Promotes normal red-blood-cell formation
- Helps in energy production
- Acts as coenzyme (see Glossary) in carbohydrate, protein and fat metabolism
- Treats some forms of anemia
- Treats cycloserine and isoniazid poisoning
- Maintains normal homocysteine levels
- Acts as a tranquilizer

 ## Possible Additional Benefits

- May promote normal nerve and muscle function
- May lower blood cholesterol
- May reduce inflammation associated with arthritis and carpal-tunnel syndrome
- Possible arteriosclerosis prevention in people with high homocysteine levels
- May reduce symptoms of premenstrual syndrome
- Potential asthmatic symptom reduction
- May promote ease in sleep by increasing serotonin

 ## Who May Benefit from Additional Amounts?

- Anyone with inadequate caloric or nutritional dietary intake or increased nutritional requirements
- Pregnant or breastfeeding women
- Those who abuse alcohol or other drugs
- People with a chronic wasting illness
- Those under excess stress for long periods
- Women taking oral contraceptives or estrogen
- People with hyperthyroidism
- People with elevated homocysteine levels

Deficiency Symptoms

Symptoms of vitamin-B-6 deficiency are nonspecific and hard to reproduce experimentally.

- Weakness
- Mental confusion
- Irritability
- Nervousness
- Insomnia
- Poor walking coordination
- Hyperactivity
- Abnormal electroencephalogram
- Anemia
- Skin lesions
- Tongue discoloration
- Muscle twitching

Usage Information

What this vitamin does:

- Acts as coenzyme (see Glossary) for metabolic functions affecting protein, carbohydrates and fat utilization
- Promotes conversion of tryptophan to niacin or serotonin

Miscellaneous information:

Avoid cooking foods that contain vitamin B-6 in large amounts of water.

Available as:

- Tablets: Swallow whole with a full glass of liquid. Don't chew or crush. Take with or 1 to 1-1/2 hours after meals unless otherwise directed by your doctor.
- Extended-release capsules or tablets: Swallow whole with a full glass of liquid. Don't chew or crush. Take with food or immediately after eating to decrease stomach irritation.
- Vitamin B-6 is a constituent of many multivitamin/mineral preparations and B-complex vitamins.

Warnings and Precautions

Don't take if you:

Are allergic to vitamin B-6.

Consult your doctor if you have:

- Been under severe stress with illness, burns, an accident, recent surgery
- Intestinal problems
- Liver disease
- Overactive thyroid
- Sickle-cell disease

Over 55:

Are more likely to have marginal deficiency.

Pregnancy:

Don't take doses greater than DRI. Large doses can cause pyridoxine dependency syndrome in the child.

Breastfeeding:

Megadoses (greater than DRI) can cause dangerous side effects in the infant.

Effect on lab tests:

May produce false-positive results in urobilinogen determinations using Ehrlich's reagent.

Storage:

- Store in a cool, dry place away from direct light, but don't freeze.
- Store safely out of reach of children.
- Don't store in bathroom medicine cabinet. Heat and moisture may change the action of the vitamin.

Others:

Regular B-6 supplements are recommended if you take chloramphenicol, cycloserine, ethionamide, hydralazine, immunosuppressants, isoniazid or penicillamine. These decrease pyridoxine absorption and can cause anemia or tingling and numbness in hands and feet.

VITAMINS

Overdose/Toxicity

- B-6 is toxic at high doses (100-250 times RDA), causing reversible nerve damage.
- Excess can cause increased oxalate in urine, leading to stone formation.

Signs and symptoms:

Clumsiness, numbness in hands and feet

What to do:

For symptoms of overdose:
Discontinue vitamin and consult doctor. Also see *Adverse Reactions or Side Effects* section below.

For accidental overdose (such as child taking entire bottle): Dial 911 (emergency), 0 for operator or call your nearest Poison Control Center.

Adverse Reactions or Side Effects

Reaction or effect	What to do
Depression when taken with oral contraceptive pills	Discontinue pyridoxine. Call doctor when convenient.
Doses of 200mg/day can produce dependency, causing need to continue to take high doses (undesirable)	Discontinue doses greater than DRI gradually.
Large doses (2 to 6 g/day) taken for several months are reported to cause severe sensory neuropathy (see Glossary) with unsteady gait, numb feet and hands, clumsiness	Discontinue doses greater than DRI. Call doctor immediately.

Interaction with Medicine, Minerals or Vitamins

Interacts with	Combined effect
Chloramphenicol, cycloserine, ethionamide, hydralazine, isoniazid, penicillamine, and immuno-suppressants (such as ACTH, adreno-corticoids, azathioprine, chlorambucil, cyclophosphamide, cyclosporine, mercaptopurine)	May increase excretion of pyridoxine and cause anemia or peripheral neuritis, which includes pain and numbness and coldness in feet and fingertips. If you take these medicines, you may need increased pyridoxine. Consult your doctor.
Estrogen or oral contraceptives	May increase requirements of pyridoxine and cause depression. Consult doctor.
Levodopa	Prevents levodopa from controlling symptoms of Parkinson's disease. This problem does not occur with carbidopa-levodopa combination.
Phenytoin	Large doses of B-6 hasten breakdown of phenytoin.

Interaction with Other Substances

Tobacco decreases absorption. Smokers may require supplemental vitamin B-6.

Lab Tests to Detect Deficiency

- Pyridoxine level in blood
- Xanthurenic-acid level in urine

Riboflavin (Vitamin B-2)

 ## Basic Information

- Available from natural sources? Yes
- Available from synthetic sources? Yes
- Prescription required? No
- Water-soluble
- *Optimal Intake,* see pages 182–183

 ## Natural Sources

Bananas	Ham
Beef liver	Mixed vegetables
Dairy products	Pork
Eggs	Tuna
Enriched breads	Wheat germ
Fortified cereals	

 ## Benefits

- Aids release of energy from food
- Maintains healthy mucous membranes lining respiratory, digestive, circulatory and excretory tracts when used in conjunction with vitamin A
- Preserves integrity of nervous system, skin, eyes
- Promotes normal growth and development
- Activates vitamin B-6
- Essential for conversion of tryptophan to niacin

 ## Possible Additional Benefits

- May increase body growth during normal developmental stages
- Possible treatment for cheilitis

 ## Who May Benefit from Additional Amounts?

- Anyone with inadequate caloric or nutritional dietary intake or increased nutritional requirements
- Pregnant or breastfeeding women
- Those who abuse alcohol or other drugs
- People with a chronic wasting illness
- Those under excess stress for long periods
- Anyone who has recently undergone surgery
- Athletes and workers who participate in vigorous physical activities
- People who have hyperthyroidism

 ## Deficiency Symptoms

- Cracks and sores in corners of mouth
- Inflammation of tongue and lips
- Eyes overly sensitive to light and easily tired
- Itching and scaling of skin around nose, mouth, scrotum, forehead, ears, scalp
- Trembling
- Insomnia

 ## Usage Information

What this vitamin does:

- Acts as component in two coenzymes (see Glossary)—flavin mononucleotide and flavin adenine dinucleotide—needed for normal tissue respiration
- Activates pyridoxine
- Works in conjunction with other B vitamins

VITAMINS

➔

Miscellaneous information:
- A balanced diet prevents deficiency without supplements.
- Large doses may produce dark yellow urine.
- Processing food may decrease quantity of vitamin B-2.
- Mixing with baking soda destroys riboflavin.
- Exposure to sunlight destroys riboflavin. Store milk in colored plastic jugs or cardboard containers.

Available as:
- Tablets: Swallow whole with a full glass of liquid. Don't chew or crush. Take with food or immediately after eating to decrease stomach irritation.
- Riboflavin is a constituent of many multivitamin/mineral preparations and B-complex vitamins.

 Warnings and Precautions

Don't take if you:
- Are allergic to any B vitamin
- Have chronic kidney failure

Consult your doctor if you are:
Pregnant or planning a pregnancy.

Over 55:
Have a greater need for vitamin B-2.

Pregnancy:
Don't take doses greater than DRI.

Breastfeeding:
Don't take doses greater than DRI.

Effect on lab tests:
- Urinary catecholamine concentration may show false elevation.
- Urobilinogen determinations (Ehrlich's) may produce false-positive results.

Storage:
- Store in a cool, dry place away from direct light, but don't freeze.
- Store safely out of reach of children.
- Don't store in bathroom medicine cabinet. Heat and moisture may change the action of the vitamin.

 Overdose/Toxicity

Vitamin B-2 is unlikely to cause toxic symptoms in healthy people with normal kidney function.

What to do:
For accidental overdose (such as child taking entire bottle): Dial 911 (emergency), 0 for operator or call your nearest Poison Control Center.

 Adverse Reactions or Side Effects

Reaction or effect	What to do
Bright yellow urine (with large doses)	No action is necessary.

 Interaction with Medicine, Minerals or Vitamins

Interacts with	Combined effect
Antidepressants (tricyclic)	Decreases B-2 effect.
Phenothiazines	Decreases B-2 effect.
Probenecid	Decreases B-2 effect.

 Interaction with Other Substances

Tobacco decreases absorption. Smokers may require supplemental vitamin B-2.

Alcohol prevents uptake and absorption of vitamin B-2.

 Lab Tests to Detect Deficiency

- Serum riboflavin
- Erythrocyte riboflavin
- Glutathione reductase

Thiamine (Vitamin B-1)

Basic Information

- Available from natural sources? Yes
- Available from synthetic sources? Yes
- Prescription required? Yes, for injectable forms
- Water-soluble
- *Optimal Intake,* see pages 182–183

Natural Sources

Baked potato	Orange juice
Beef kidney/liver	Oranges
Brewer's yeast	Oysters
Flour, rye and whole grain	Peanuts
	Peas
Garbanzo beans (chickpeas), dried	Raisins
	Rice, brown and raw
Ham	Wheat germ
Kidney beans, dried	Whole-grain products
Navy beans, dried	

Benefits

- Keeps mucous membranes healthy
- Maintains normal function of nervous system, muscles, heart
- Aids in treatment of herpes zoster
- Promotes normal growth and development
- Treats beriberi (thiamine-deficiency disease)
- Replaces deficiency caused by alcoholism, cirrhosis, overactive thyroid, infection, breastfeeding, absorption diseases, pregnancy, prolonged diarrhea, burns

Possible Additional Benefits

- May reduce depression
- May reduce fatigue
- May reduce motion sickness
- May improve appetite and mental alertness

Who May Benefit from Additional Amounts?

- People who abuse alcohol or other drugs (Alcoholics need more thiamine. Thiamine accelerates metabolism, using extra carbohydrates and calories from alcohol.)
- Anyone with inadequate caloric or nutritional dietary intake or increased nutritional requirements
- People over 55 years old
- Pregnant or breastfeeding women
- People with a chronic wasting illness, especially diabetes
- Those under excess stress for long periods
- Anyone who has recently undergone surgery
- People with liver disease, overactive thyroid, prolonged diarrhea

Deficiency Symptoms

Normal deficiency:
- Loss of appetite
- Fatigue
- Nausea
- Mental problems, such as rolling of eyeballs, depression, memory loss, difficulty concentrating and dealing

VITAMINS

➜

with details, personality changes, rapid heartbeat
- Gastrointestinal disorders
- Tender, atrophied muscles
- Wernicke's encephalopathy

Gross deficiency:
- Leads eventually to beriberi, which is rare except in severely ill alcoholics
- Pain or tingling in arms or legs
- Decreased reflex activity
- Fluid accumulation in arms and legs
- Heart enlargement
- Constipation
- Nausea
- Vomiting

Usage Information

What this vitamin does:

Thiamine functions in combination with adenosine triphosphate to form coenzyme (see Glossary) necessary for converting carbohydrates into energy in muscles and nervous system.

Miscellaneous information:
- Cook foods in minimum amount of water or steam.
- Avoid high cooking temperatures and long heat exposure.
- Avoid using baking soda when you take thiamine unless it is used as a leavening agent in baked products.
- Thiamine is stable when frozen and stored.
- A balanced diet should provide enough thiamine for healthy people to make supplementation unnecessary. The best dietary sources of thiamine are whole-grain cereals and meat.

Available as:
- Tablets: Swallow whole with a full glass of liquid. Don't chew or crush. Take with or 1 to 1-1/2 hours after meals unless otherwise directed by your doctor.

- Liquid: Dilute in at least 1/2 glass of water or other liquid. Take with or 1 to 1-1/2 hours after meals unless otherwise directed by your doctor.
- Injectable forms are administered by a doctor or nurse.
- Available as part of B complex.

Warnings and Precautions

Don't take if you:
Are allergic to any B vitamin.

Consult your doctor if you have:
Liver or kidney disease.

Pregnancy:
Don't take doses greater than DRI.

Breastfeeding:
Don't take doses greater than DRI.

Effect on lab tests:
Interferes with results of serum theophyline and may produce false-positive results in tests for uric acid or urobilinogen.

Storage:
- Store in a cool, dry place away from direct light, but don't freeze.
- Store safely out of reach of children.
- Don't store in bathroom medicine cabinet. Heat and moisture may change the action of the vitamin.

Others:
Most excess thiamine is excreted in urine if kidney function is normal.

Overdose/Toxicity

Signs and symptoms:

Occasionally large doses of vitamin B-1 have caused hypersensitive reactions resembling anaphylactic shock. Several hundred milligrams may cause drowsiness in some people.

What to do:

For symptoms of overdose:

Discontinue vitamin and consult doctor. Also see *Adverse Reactions or Side Effects* section below.

For accidental overdose (such as child taking entire bottle): Dial 911 (emergency), 0 for operator or call your nearest Poison Control Center.

Adverse Reactions or Side Effects

Reaction or effect	What to do
Skin rash or itching (rare)	Discontinue. Call doctor immediately.
Swelling in facial area	Discontinue. Call doctor immediately.
Wheezing (more likely after intravenous dose)	Seek emergency treatment.

Interaction with Medicine, Minerals or Vitamins

Interacts with	Combined effect
Antibiotics or sulfa drugs	Decreases thiamine levels.
Drugs used to relax muscles during surgery	Produces excessive muscle relaxation. Tell your doctor before surgery if you are taking supplements.

Oral contraceptives	Decreases thiamine levels.
Wernicke's encephalopathy treatment	Take thiamine before taking glucose.

Interaction with Other Substances

Tobacco decreases absorption. Smokers may require supplemental vitamin B-1.

Alcohol reduces intestinal absorption of vitamin B-1, which is necessary to metabolize alcohol.

Beverages:

Carbonates and citrates (additives listed on many beverage labels) decrease thiamine effect.

Foods:

Carbonates and citrates (additives listed on many food labels) decrease thiamine effect.

Lab Tests to Detect Deficiency

• Transketolase function study on red blood cells
• Pyruvic-acid blood level
• 24-hour urine collection

VITAMINS

Amino Acids and Nucleic Acids

Amino Acids

Amino acids are a chemical group containing nitrogen, carbon, oxygen and hydrogen. The amino acids form the chief structure of proteins, several of which are essential for human growth, development and nutrition.

Supplementation with commercially available forms should not be necessary.

Nucleic Acids

These chemicals contain sugars, phosphoric acid, purines and pyrimidine bases (see Glossary). The two most studied nucleic acids are chemicals found in the genes: ribonucleic acid (RNA) and deoxyribonucleic acid (DNA) (see Glossary). Nucleic acids taken as supplements have little or no value. Nucleic acids taken as injections can be dangerous.

Arginine

Basic Information

Arginine is an amino acid.

- Available from natural sources? Yes
- Available from synthetic sources? Yes
- Prescription required? No

Natural Sources

Brown rice	Popcorn
Carob	Raisins
Chocolate	Raw cereals
Nuts	Sesame seeds
Oatmeal	Sunflower seeds
Peanuts/peanut butter	Whole-wheat products

Benefits

- Functions as building block of all proteins
- Stimulates human-growth hormone
- Stimulates immune system
- Helps treat HIV infection by boosting activity of immune-system fighting cells
- Used to treat liver disorders
- Increases metabolism in fat cells to decrease obesity
- Builds muscle
- Speeds wound healing

Possible Additional Benefits

May inhibit cancer and growth of tumors

Who May Benefit from Additional Amounts?

- Those with inadequate protein dietary intake
- Children and pregnant or breastfeeding women who are vegan vegetarians
- People with recent severe burns or injuries
- Premature infants
- People with diseases that suppress the immune system, such as AIDS

Deficiency Symptoms

Single amino-acid deficiencies are unknown except in people on crash diets consisting of only a few foods. Amino-acid deficiencies appear more commonly as a result of total protein deficiency, which is rare in the United States and Canada.

- Impaired insulin production
- Impaired liver-lipid metabolism

Usage Information

What this amino acid does:

- Provides part of all proteins
- Stimulates activity and size of thymus gland, causing it to increase production of cells that are crucial to the immune system

Miscellaneous information:

- Arginine has been reported to increase the activity of some herpes viruses and inhibit others.
- Arginine competes with lysine for absorption.

Available as:

• Tablets or capsules: Follow manufacturer's instructions unless otherwise recommended by your doctor.

• Powder for oral solution: Dissolve powder in cold water or juice. Take with or 1 to 1-1/2 hours after meals unless otherwise directed by your doctor.

Warnings and Precautions

Don't take if you are:

• A child or adolescent not fully grown

• Allergic to any food protein, such as eggs, milk, wheat

• At risk of poor nutrition for any reason

Consult your doctor if you:

Have any bone disease.

Over 55:

Don't take amino-acid supplements if you are healthy.

Pregnancy:

Don't take amino-acid supplements.

Breastfeeding:

Don't take amino-acid supplements.

Storage:

• Store in cool, dry place away from direct light, but don't freeze.

• Store safely out of reach of children.

• Don't store in bathroom medicine cabinet. Heat and moisture may change the action of the amino acid.

Others:

Children and adolescents should not take any arginine supplement. It may cause bone deformities.

Overdose/Toxicity

Signs and symptoms:

Unlikely to threaten life or cause significant symptoms.

What to do:

For symptoms of overdose:

Discontinue amino acid and consult doctor. Also see *Adverse Reactions or Side Effects* section below.

For accidental overdose (such as child taking entire bottle): Dial 911 (emergency), 0 for operator or call your nearest Poison Control Center.

Adverse Reactions or Side Effects

Note: Impurities in amino-acid supplements have resulted in diverse health problems.

Reaction or effect	What to do
Diarrhea (from large doses)	Decrease dose or discontinue.
Nausea (from large doses)	Decrease dose or discontinue.

Interaction with Medicine, Minerals or Vitamins

None are known.

Lab Tests to Detect Deficiency

None are available, except for experimental purposes.

Glutamine

 Basic Information

Glutamine converts to the amino acid called *glutamic acid.*

- Available from natural sources? Yes
- Available from synthetic sources? Yes
- Prescription required? No

 Natural Sources

Raw parsley
Spinach

 Benefits

- Functions as building block of all proteins
- Aids digestive tract
- Important for muscle growth and maintenance
- Decreases muscle wasting
- Enhances digestive-system function in trauma patients and cancer patients on chemotherapy

 Possible Additional Benefits

- May treat intestinal disorders and peptic ulcers
- Possible treatment for connective-tissue diseases and damage to tissue from radiation treatment
- May enhance brain function and mental activity by boosting GABA (gamma-aminobutyric acid) levels (see Glossary)

 Who May Benefit from Additional Amounts?

- Those with inadequate protein dietary intake
- People who experience muscle wasting due to disease (such as cancer or AIDS) or lengthy bed rest
- Trauma patients or patients on high-dose chemotherapy such as bone marrow–transplant patients

 Deficiency Symptoms

Single amino-acid deficiencies are unknown except in people on crash diets consisting of only a few foods. Amino-acid deficiencies appear more commonly as a result of total protein deficiency, which is rare in the United States and Canada.

 Usage Information

What this amino acid does:

- Converts into glutamic acid when it passes through the blood-brain barrier (Glutamic acid is critical for cerebral function.)
- Participates in regulating the proper acid/alkaline balance
- Participates in the synthesis of RNA and DNA (see Glossary)

Miscellaneous information:

- Poorly nourished people have a greater chance of adverse side effects from taking amino-acid supplements, including an amino-acid imbalance.
- Muscles contain large amounts of glutamine.

• Glutamine is considered a non-essential amino acid; however, recent findings indicate that in high-stress situations, such as trauma, it may be essential.

Available as:

Powder: Follow manufacturer's instructions.

Warnings and Precautions

Don't take if you have:
• Kidney problems
• Cirrhosis of the liver
• Reye's syndrome

Consult your doctor if you:

Are undergoing chemotherapy.

Over 55:

Don't take amino-acid supplements if you are healthy.

Pregnancy:

Don't take amino-acid supplements.

Breastfeeding:

Don't take amino-acid supplements.

Storage:
• Store safely out of reach of children.
• Don't store in bathroom medicine cabinet. Heat and moisture may change the action of the amino acid.
• Keep the supplement completely dry or the quality will deteriorate.

Others:

It is best to consume complete proteins rather than individual amino acids.

Overdose/Toxicity

Signs and symptoms:
• May decrease production of growth hormone
• Decreases bicarbonate buffer (which may upset the acid-base balance of the stomach)

What to do:

For symptoms of overdose:
Discontinue amino acid and consult doctor.

For accidental overdose (such as child taking entire bottle): Dial 911 (emergency), 0 for operator or call your nearest Poison Control Center.

Adverse Reactions or Side Effects

None are expected.

Interaction with Medicine, Minerals or Vitamins

None are expected.

Lab Tests to Detect Deficiency

None are available, except for experimental purposes.

AMINO ACIDS

L-Cysteine

Basic Information

L-cysteine is an amino acid.

- Available from natural sources? Yes
- Available from synthetic sources? Yes
- Prescription required? No

Natural Sources

Cereals (some)
Dairy products
Eggs
Meat
Whole grains

Benefits

- Functions as building block of all proteins
- Eliminates certain toxic chemicals, rendering them harmless (antioxidant—see Glossary)

Possible Additional Benefits

- Contains sulfur in a form believed to inactivate free radicals—if so, it protects and preserves cells
- May help build muscle
- May burn fat
- May protect against toxins and pollutants, including some found in cigarette smoke and alcohol
- May combat arthritis
- May participate in some forms of DNA (see Glossary) repair and theoretically extend life span
- Potential aid in treatment of respiratory disorders
- May slow viral replication in HIV
- May help treat asthma when inhaled in mist form

Who May Benefit from Additional Amounts?

- Those with inadequate protein dietary intake
- Children and pregnant or breast-feeding women who are vegan vegetarians
- People with recent severe burns or injuries
- Premature infants

Deficiency Symptoms

Single amino-acid deficiencies are unknown except in people on crash diets consisting of only a few foods. Amino-acid deficiencies appear more commonly as a result of total protein deficiency, which is rare in the United States and Canada.

Moderate deficiency:

- Slowed growth in children
- Low levels of essential proteins in blood

Severe deficiency:

- Apathy
- Depigmentation of hair
- Edema (excess fluid in connective tissue)
- Lethargy
- Liver damage
- Loss of muscle and fat
- Skin lesions
- Weakness

Usage Information

What this amino acid does:
- Provides part of all proteins
- Functions in synthesis of glutathione, a substance that may neutralize environmental pollutants, including tobacco

Miscellaneous information:
- Poorly nourished people have a greater chance of adverse side effects from taking amino-acid supplements, including an amino-acid imbalance.
- Take L-cysteine supplements with vitamin C. Take 2 to 3 times as much vitamin C as cysteine, milligram to milligram, as a precaution against kidney- or bladder-stone formation.
- L-cysteine is used under medical supervision in emergency rooms to protect against liver damage caused by overdoses of acetaminophen.

Available as:
Capsules: Swallow whole with a full glass of liquid. Don't chew or crush. Take with or 1 to 1-1/2 hours after meals unless otherwise directed by your doctor.

Warnings and Precautions

Don't take if you are:
- Allergic to any food protein, such as eggs, milk, wheat
- Diabetic
- Self-prescribing without medical supervision

Consult your doctor if you have:
- Diabetes mellitus
- Cystinuria

Over 55:
Don't take amino-acid supplements if you are healthy.

Pregnancy:
Don't take amino-acid supplements.

Breastfeeding:
Don't take amino-acid supplements.

Storage:
- Store in cool, dry place away from direct light, but don't freeze.
- Store safely out of reach of children.
- Don't store in bathroom medicine cabinet. Heat and moisture may change the action of the amino acid.

Overdose/Toxicity

Signs and symptoms:
Unlikely to threaten life or cause significant symptoms.

What to do:

For symptoms of overdose:
Discontinue amino acid and consult doctor.

For accidental overdose (such as child taking entire bottle): Dial 911 (emergency), 0 for operator or call your nearest Poison Control Center.

Adverse Reactions or Side Effects
None are expected.

Interaction with Medicine, Minerals or Vitamins

Interacts with	Combined effect
Insulin	May inactivate insulin effect.

AMINO ACIDS

→

Monosodium-glutamate (MSG)	L-cysteine may increase toxicity of monosodium glutamate in individuals who suffer from the "Chinese-restaurant syndrome." Causes headache, dizziness, disorientation and burning sensations.
Vitamin C	Taken with L-cysteine, vitamin C helps prevent L-cysteine from converting to cystine, which may cause bladder or kidney stones.

 Lab Tests to Detect Deficiency

None are available, except for experimental purposes.

L-Lysine

 Basic Information

L-lysine is an amino acid.

- Available from natural sources? Yes
- Available from synthetic sources? Yes
- Prescription required? No

 Natural Sources

Cheese	Potatoes
Eggs	Red meat
Fish	Soy products
Lima beans	Yeast
Milk	

 Benefits

- Functions as essential building block of all proteins
- Promotes growth, tissue repair and production of antibodies, hormones, enzymes

 Possible Additional Benefits

- May protect against herpes viruses
- May prevent recurrence of cold sores and lessen severity of outbreaks

 Who May Benefit from Additional Amounts?

- Those with inadequate protein dietary intake
- Children and pregnant or breastfeeding women who are vegan vegetarians

 Deficiency Symptoms

Single amino-acid deficiencies are unknown except in people on crash diets consisting of only a few foods. Amino-acid deficiencies appear more commonly as a result of total protein deficiency, which is rare in the United States and Canada.

Moderate deficiency:
- Slowed growth in children
- Low levels of essential proteins in blood

Severe deficiency:
- Apathy
- Depigmentation of hair
- Edema (excess fluid in connective tissue)
- Lethargy
- Liver damage
- Loss of muscle and fat
- Skin lesions
- Weakness

Usage Information

What this amino acid does:
- L-lysine is one of eight essential amino acids that the body does not manufacture.
- All biological amino acids participate in the synthesis of proteins in animal bodies.

Miscellaneous information:
- There is no scientific evidence to show that supplements are needed or helpful.
- Poorly nourished people have a greater chance of adverse side effects from taking amino-acid supplements, including an amino-acid imbalance.
- L-lysine competes with arginine for absorption.

Available as:
- Capsules: Swallow whole with a full glass of liquid. Don't chew or crush. Take with or 1 to 1-1/2 hours after meals unless otherwise directed by your doctor.
- Lysine is a constituent of many multivitamin/mineral preparations.

Warnings and Precautions

Don't take if you are:
- Allergic to any food protein, such as eggs, milk, wheat

- At risk of poor nutrition for any reason
- Self-prescribing without medical supervision

Consult your doctor if you:
Have diabetes mellitus.

Over 55:
Don't take amino-acid supplements if you are healthy.

Pregnancy:
Don't take amino-acid supplements.

Breastfeeding:
Don't take amino-acid supplements.

None are known.

Storage:
- Store in cool, dry place away from direct light, but don't freeze.
- Store safely out of reach of children.
- Don't store in bathroom medicine cabinet. Heat and moisture may change the action of the amino acid.

Overdose/Toxicity

Signs and symptoms:
Unlikely to threaten life or cause significant symptoms.

What to do:
For symptoms of overdose:
Discontinue amino acid and consult doctor.

For accidental overdose (such as child taking entire bottle): Dial 911 (emergency), 0 for operator or call your nearest Poison Control Center.

Adverse Reactions or Side Effects

None are expected.

→

AMINO ACIDS

Interaction with Medicine, Minerals or Vitamins

None are expected.

Interaction with Other Substances

Foods high in arginine (nuts, chocolate, seeds, carob and raisins) decrease the ability of L-lysine to prevent or reduce cold sore outbreaks.

Lab Tests to Detect Deficiency

None are available, except for experimental purposes.

Methionine

Basic Information

Methionine is an amino acid. S-adenosyl-methionine (SAM), a by-product of methionine, is more widely used in Europe.

• Available from natural sources? Yes
• Available from synthetic sources? Yes
• Prescription required? No

Natural Sources

Beans	Lentils
Eggs	Meat
Fish	Milk
Garlic	Onions

Benefits

Functions as building block of all proteins

Possible Additional Benefits

• May be effective adjuvant treatment for depression—consult doctor
• Cysteine and taurine may rely on methionine for synthesis in the human body

Who May Benefit from Additional Amounts?

• Those with inadequate protein dietary intake
• Vegan vegetarians
• People with recent severe burns or injuries
• Premature infants

Deficiency Symptoms

Single amino-acid deficiencies are unknown except in people on crash diets consisting of only a few foods. Amino-acid deficiencies appear more commonly as a result of total protein deficiency, which is rare in the United States and Canada.

Moderate deficiency:
- Slowed growth in children
- Low levels of essential proteins in blood

Severe deficiency:
- Apathy
- Depigmentation of hair
- Edema (excess fluid in connective tissue)
- Lethargy
- Liver damage
- Loss of muscle and fat
- Skin lesions
- Weakness

Usage Information

What this amino acid does:
Methionine provides part of all proteins.

Miscellaneous information:
- This sulfur-containing amino acid (like choline and taurine) may help eliminate fatty substances that could cause occlusion (see Glossary) of vital arteries.
- Poorly nourished people have a greater chance of adverse side effects from taking amino-acid supplements, including an amino-acid imbalance.
- Few people need methionine supplements.

Available as:
- Tablets: Swallow whole with a full glass of liquid. Don't chew or crush. Take with or 1 to 1-1/2 hours after meals unless otherwise directed by your doctor.
- Capsules: Swallow whole with a full glass of liquid. Don't chew or crush. Take with food or immediately after eating to decrease stomach irritation.

Warnings and Precautions

Don't take if you are:
- Allergic to any food protein, such as eggs, milk, wheat
- At risk of poor nutrition for any reason

Consult your doctor if you:
Self-prescribed methionine without medical supervision.

Over 55:
Don't take amino-acid supplements if you are healthy.

Pregnancy:
Don't take amino-acid supplements.

Breastfeeding:
Don't take amino-acid supplements.

Storage:
- Store in cool, dry place away from direct light, but don't freeze.
- Store safely out of reach of children.
- Don't store in bathroom medicine cabinet. Heat and moisture may change the action of the amino acid.

Overdose/Toxicity

Signs and symptoms:
Unlikely to threaten life or cause significant symptoms.

What to do:
For symptoms of overdose:
Discontinue amino acid and consult doctor.

For accidental overdose (such as child taking entire bottle): Dial 911 (emergency), 0 for operator or call your nearest Poison Control Center.

AMINO ACIDS

→

Adverse Reactions or Side Effects

None are expected.

Interaction with Medicine, Minerals or Vitamins

None are known.

Lab Tests to Detect Deficiency

None are available, except for experimental purposes.

Phenylalanine

Basic Information

Phenylalanine is an amino acid.

• Available from natural sources? Yes
• Available from synthetic sources? Yes
• Prescription required? No

Natural Sources

Almonds	Peanuts
Avocados	Pickled herring
Bananas	Pumpkin seeds
Cheese	Sesame seeds
Cottage cheese	Sugar products with
Lima beans	aspartame
Nonfat dried milk	

Benefits

• Functions as building block of all proteins
• Can induce significant short-term increases of blood levels of norepinephrine, dopamine and epinephrine, which may be harmful at times and helpful at others (Don't take without medical supervision!)

Possible Additional Benefits

No proven additional benefits exist.

Who May Benefit from Additional Amounts?

• Those with inadequate protein dietary intake
• Children and pregnant or breastfeeding women who are vegan vegetarians
• People with recent severe burns or injuries
• Premature infants

Deficiency Symptoms

Single amino-acid deficiencies are unknown except in people on crash diets consisting of only a few foods. Amino-acid deficiencies appear more commonly as a result of total protein deficiency, which is rare in the United States and Canada.

Moderate deficiency:
• Slowed growth in children
• Low levels of essential proteins in blood

Severe deficiency:
• Apathy
• Depigmentation of hair

- Edema (excess fluid in connective tissue)
- Lethargy
- Liver damage
- Loss of muscle and fat
- Skin lesions
- Weakness

Usage Information

What this amino acid does:

It is involved in the production of dopamine and epinephrine, which affect transmission of impulses in the human brain and other parts of the nervous system.

Miscellaneous information:

- Supplements taken by healthy people will not make them healthier.
- Poorly nourished people have a greater chance of adverse side effects from taking amino-acid supplements, including an amino-acid imbalance.

Available as:

- Tablets: Swallow whole with a full glass of liquid. Don't chew or crush. Take with or 1 to 1-1/2 hours after meals unless otherwise directed by your doctor.
- There are three different forms of phenylalanine: L, D and D L. The most common type is L. Consult your doctor about the proper type for you.

Warnings and Precautions

Don't take if you:

- Are allergic to any food protein, such as eggs, milk, wheat
- Are at risk of poor nutrition for any reason
- Suffer from migraine headaches
- Have phenylketonuria (PKU)
- Have pigmented malignant melanoma, a deadly form of skin cancer
- Take any monoamine oxidase inhibitor as an antidepressant, including pargyline, isocarboxazid, phenelzine, procarbazine, tranylcypromine
- Have diabetes
- Are pregnant
- Suffer from anxiety attacks

Consult your doctor if you:

- Have high blood pressure
- Self-medicated with phenylalanine for any reason without medical supervision

Over 55:

Don't take amino-acid supplements if you are healthy.

Pregnancy:

- Don't take amino-acid supplements.
- Pregnant women and children with PKU must follow a phenylalanine-free or -low diet to maintain health. Consult your doctor.

Breastfeeding:

Don't take amino-acid supplements.

Storage:

- Store in cool, dry place away from direct light, but don't freeze.
- Store safely out of reach of children.
- Don't store in bathroom medicine cabinet. Heat and moisture may change the action of the amino acid.

Others:

- Phenylalanine may cause high blood pressure to rise even higher.
- It can cause mental retardation in children with PKU.

AMINO ACIDS

→

Overdose/Toxicity

Signs and symptoms:
Unlikely to threaten life or cause significant symptoms.

What to do:
For symptoms of overdose:
Discontinue amino acid and consult doctor. Also see *Adverse Reactions or Side Effects* section below.

For accidental overdose (such as child taking entire bottle): Dial 911 (emergency), 0 for operator or call your nearest Poison Control Center.

 Adverse Reactions or Side Effects

Reaction or effect	What to do
Lowers blood pressure	Discontinue. Call doctor immediately.
Migraine headaches	Discontinue. Call doctor immediately.
Raises blood pressure	Discontinue. Call doctor immediately.

 Interaction with Medicine, Minerals or Vitamins

Interacts with	Combined effect
Antidepressant drugs (containing monoamine oxidase inhibitors)	Dangerous or life-threatening blood-pressure elevation.
Tyrosine	Additive effect with phenylalanine greatly increases chance of undesirable side effects.

 Lab Tests to Detect Deficiency

None are available, except for experimental purposes.

Serine

 Basic Information

Serine is an amino acid.

• Available from natural sources? Yes
• Available from synthetic sources? Yes
• Prescription required? No

 Natural Sources

Dairy products
Meat
Peanuts
Soy
Wheat gluten

Benefits

- Functions as building block of all proteins
- Aids metabolism of fats
- Important for muscle growth and maintenance
- Used in skin care products as a natural moisturizer

Possible Additional Benefits

None are known.

Who May Benefit from Additional Amounts?

Anyone with inadequate caloric or nutritional dietary intake or increased nutritional requirements

Deficiency Symptoms

Single amino-acid deficiencies are unknown except in people on crash diets consisting of only a few foods. Amino-acid deficiencies appear more commonly as a result of total protein deficiency, which is rare in the United States and Canada.

Usage Information

What this amino acid does:
Serine helps produce antibodies.

Miscellaneous information:
- Poorly nourished people have a greater chance of adverse side effects

from taking amino-acid supplements, including an amino-acid imbalance.
- Serine is considered a nonessential amino acid.

Available as:
A constituent of some amino-acid supplements.

Warnings and Precautions

Don't take if you are:
- Allergic to any food protein, such as eggs, milk, wheat
- Self-prescribing without medical supervision

Consult your doctor if you are:
Considering taking serine.

Over 55:
Don't take amino-acid supplements if you are healthy.

Pregnancy:
Don't take amino-acid supplements.

Breastfeeding:
Don't take amino-acid supplements.

Storage:
- Store in cool, dry place away from direct light, but don't freeze.
- Store safely out of reach of children.
- Don't store in bathroom medicine cabinet. Heat and moisture may change the action of the amino acid.

Overdose/Toxicity

What to do:
For symptoms of overdose:
Discontinue amino acid and consult doctor.

AMINO ACIDS

→

For accidental overdose (such as child taking entire bottle): Dial 911 (emergency), 0 for operator or call your nearest Poison Control Center.

 Adverse Reactions or Side Effects

None are expected.

 Interaction with Medicine, Minerals or Vitamins

None are known.

 Lab Tests to Detect Deficiency

None are available, except for experimental purposes.

Taurine

 Basic Information

Taurine is an amino acid that is *nonessential*—it can be made by the body.

- Available from natural sources? Yes
- Available from synthetic sources? Yes
- Prescription required? No

 Natural Sources

Breast milk
Eggs
Fish (especially clams and oysters)
Meat
Milk
Note: Taurine is not available from plant sources.

 Benefits

Helps regulate fluid balance

 Possible Additional Benefits

- May stabilize heart rhythm
- May contribute to antioxidant (see Glossary) defense
- May be essential for growth of infants, children, adolescents
- May strengthen heart muscle
- May reduce Adriamycin toxicity
- May help control high blood pressure
- May reduce platelet clumping

 Who May Benefit from Additional Amounts?

- Those with inadequate protein dietary intake
- Children and pregnant or breast-feeding women who are vegan vegetarians
- People with recent severe burns or injuries
- Premature infants

Deficiency Symptoms

Single amino-acid deficiencies are unknown except in people on crash diets consisting of only a few foods. Amino-acid deficiencies appear more commonly as a result of total protein deficiency, which is rare in the United States and Canada.

Moderate deficiency:
- Slowed growth in children
- Low levels of essential proteins in blood

Severe deficiency:
- Apathy
- Depigmentation of hair
- Edema (excess fluid in connective tissue)
- Lethargy
- Liver damage
- Loss of muscle and fat
- Skin lesions
- Weakness

Usage Information

What this amino acid does:
Taurine functions in electrically active tissues, such as the brain and heart, to help stabilize cell membranes.

Miscellaneous information:
- Taurine is synthesized from methionine and cystine. Vitamin B-6 is needed for this synthesis.
- Healthy people who eat well-balanced diets don't need taurine supplements.

- Poorly nourished people have a greater chance of adverse side effects from taking amino-acid supplements, including an amino-acid imbalance.
- Breast milk is rich in taurine.

Available as:
- Tablets: Swallow whole with a full glass of liquid. Don't chew or crush. Take with or 1 to 1-1/2 hours after meals unless otherwise directed by your doctor.
- Capsules: Swallow whole with a full glass of liquid. Don't chew or crush. Take with or 1 to 1-1/2 hours after meals unless otherwise directed by your doctor.

Warnings and Precautions

Don't take if you:
- Are allergic to any food protein such as eggs, milk, wheat
- Are at risk of poor nutrition for any reason
- Have stomach ulcers

Consult your doctor if you have:
- Epilepsy
- Eye problems
- Self-prescribed taurine without medical supervision

Over 55:
Don't take amino-acid supplements if you are healthy.

Pregnancy:
Don't take amino-acid supplements.

Breastfeeding:
Don't take amino-acid supplements.

Storage:
- Store in cool, dry place away from direct light, but don't freeze.

AMINO ACIDS

- Store safely out of reach of children.
- Don't store in bathroom medicine cabinet. Heat and moisture may change the action of the amino acid.

Overdose/Toxicity

Signs and symptoms:
Unlikely to threaten life or cause significant symptoms.

What to do:
For symptoms of overdose:
Discontinue amino acid and consult doctor. Also see *Adverse Reactions or Side Effects* section below.

For accidental overdose (such as child taking entire bottle): Dial 911 (emergency), 0 for operator or call your nearest Poison Control Center.

Adverse Reactions or Side Effects

Reaction or effect	What to do
Depression of central nervous system	Discontinue. Call doctor immediately.
Memory deficits	Discontinue. Call doctor when convenient.

Interaction with Medicine, Minerals or Vitamins

Interacts with	Combined effect
Anticonvulsants	May decrease frequency of seizures.

Interaction with Other Substances

Alcohol: Excessive alcohol intake causes large urinary loss of taurine and impaired utilization of taurine.

Food and beverages: Intake of monosodium glutamate (MSG) and aspartame may reduce taurine levels.

Lab Tests to Detect Deficiency

None are available, except for experimental purposes.

Tryptophan Declared unsafe: DO NOT TAKE!

Basic Information

Tryptophan is an amino acid.

- Available from natural sources? Yes
- Available from synthetic sources? Yes
- Prescription required? No

Natural Sources

Barley
Brown rice
Cottage cheese
Fish (tuna, crab, shellfish)
Meats (beef, chicken, duck, turkey)
Milk
Peanuts
Soybeans

Note: You cannot get enough tryptophan from natural sources to cause adverse reactions.

Benefits

Functions as building block of all proteins

Possible Additional Benefits

- May reduce alcohol cravings
- May be an effective sleep aid
- Potential antidepressant
- May help treat cocaine addiction
- May decrease sensitivity to moderate pain

Who May Benefit from Additional Amounts?

- Those with inadequate protein dietary intake
- Children and pregnant or breastfeeding women who are vegan vegetarians
- People with recent severe burns or injuries
- Premature infants

Deficiency Symptoms

Single amino-acid deficiencies are unknown except in people on crash diets consisting of only a few foods. Amino-acid deficiencies appear more commonly as a result of total protein deficiency, which is rare in the United States and Canada.

Moderate deficiency:
- Slowed growth in children
- Low levels of essential proteins in blood

Severe deficiency:
- Apathy
- Depigmentation of hair
- Edema (excess fluid in connective tissue)
- Lethargy
- Liver damage
- Loss of muscle and fat
- Skin lesions
- Weakness

Usage Information

What this amino acid does:
- Provides part of all proteins
- Participates in biosynthesis of a neurotransmitter (see Glossary) called serotonin, which may induce certain stages of sleep

Miscellaneous information:

Contaminated supplements have been related to several deaths in the United States.

Available as:
- Tryptophan has been withdrawn from the United States market by the U.S. Food and Drug Administration.
- 5-hydroxytryptophan (5-HTP), a supplement that contains a form of tryptophan, is now available.

Warnings and Precautions

Don't take:

May cause eosinophilia-myalgia, a potentially fatal adverse reaction. Declared unsafe by the U.S. Food and Drug Administration and withdrawn from the U.S. market.

Consult your doctor if you:
- Take medicines to induce sleep
- Have asthma—tryptophan may increase breathing problems
- Have taken or are taking antidepressants

AMINO ACIDS

→

Over 55:
Don't take tryptophan.

Pregnancy:
Don't take tryptophan.

Breastfeeding:
Don't take tryptophan.

Storage:
Not applicable—tryptophan supplements are unavailable.

Others:
• Tryptophan has caused eosinophilia-myalgia, a potentially fatal adverse reaction. (The adverse reaction of eosinophilia-myalgia was caused by a contaminant found in supplements, not tryptophan itself.)
• In experimental studies of animals with vitamin B-6 deficiency, large doses of tryptophan caused bladder cancer.
• If you have any tryptophan in your medicine cabinet, throw it out.

 Overdose/Toxicity

Signs and symptoms:
May cause eosinophilia-myalgia, a potentially fatal adverse reaction.

What to do:
For symptoms of overdose:
Discontinue amino acid and consult doctor immediately.

For accidental overdose (such as child taking entire bottle): Dial 911 (emergency), 0 for operator or call your nearest Poison Control Center.

 Adverse Reactions or Side Effects

Tryptophan has caused eosinophilia-myalgia, a potentially fatal adverse reaction.

 Interaction with Medicine, Minerals or Vitamins

None are known.

 Lab Tests to Detect Deficiency

None are available, except for experimental purposes.

Tyrosine

Basic Information

- Available from natural sources? Yes
- Available from synthetic sources? Yes
- Prescription required? No

Natural Sources

Canned beans with pork	Lima beans
	Meat
Cheese, especially	Miso
cheddar	Peanuts
Cottage cheese	Pumpkin seeds
Eggs	Shellfish
Fish	Soybeans
Ice cream	

Benefits

- Functions as building block of all proteins
- Can induce significant short-term increases of blood levels of norepinephrine, dopamine and epinephrine, which may be harmful at times and helpful at others (Don't take without medical supervision!)

Possible Additional Benefits

- May regulate and elevate moods
- May help reduce mental depression
- May improve memory
- May diminish pain
- May increase mental alertness
- May reduce Parkinson's disease symptoms (under medical care)
- May treat chronic fatigue and narcolepsy
- May reduce stress
- May reduce body fat
- May help with withdrawal from cocaine addiction (under medical supervision)

Who May Benefit from Additional Amounts?

- Those with inadequate protein dietary intake
- Children and pregnant or breastfeeding women who are vegan vegetarians
- People with recent severe burns or injuries
- Premature infants

Deficiency Symptoms

Single amino-acid deficiencies are unknown except in people on crash diets consisting of only a few foods. Amino-acid deficiencies appear more commonly as a result of total protein deficiency, which is rare in the United States and Canada.

Moderate deficiency:
- Slowed growth in children
- Low levels of essential proteins in blood

Severe deficiency:
- Apathy
- Depigmentation of hair
- Edema (excess fluid in connective tissue)
- Lethargy
- Liver damage
- Loss of muscle and fat
- Skin lesions
- Weakness

AMINO ACIDS

Unproved speculated symptoms:
- Lack of sexual interest
- Impotence
- Poor memory
- Obesity

Usage Information

What this amino acid does:
It is involved in the production of dopamine and epinephrine, which affect transmission of impulses in the human brain and other parts of the nervous system.

Miscellaneous information:
- Supplements taken by healthy people will not make them healthier.
- Poorly nourished people have a greater chance of adverse side effects from taking amino-acid supplements, including an amino-acid imbalance.
- Take with a high carbohydrate meal or at bedtime.

Available as:
Tablets: Swallow whole with a full glass of liquid. Don't chew or crush. Take with or 1 to 1-1/2 hours after meals unless otherwise directed by your doctor.

Warnings and Precautions

Don't take if you:
- Are allergic to any food protein, such as eggs, milk, wheat
- Are at risk of poor nutrition for any reason
- Suffer from migraine headaches
- Have phenylketonuria (PKU)
- Have pigmented malignant melanoma, a deadly form of skin cancer
- Take any monamine oxidase inhibitor as an antidepressant, including pargyline, isocarboxazid, phenelzine, procarbazine, tranylcypromine

Consult your doctor if you:
- Have high blood pressure
- Self-medicated with tyrosine for any reason without medical supervision

Over 55:
Don't take amino-acid supplements if you are healthy.

Pregnancy:
Don't take amino-acid supplements.

Breastfeeding:
Don't take amino-acid supplements.

Storage:
- Store in cool, dry place away from direct light, but don't freeze.
- Store safely out of reach of children.
- Don't store in bathroom medicine cabinet. Heat and moisture may change the action of the amino acid.

Others:
Tyrosine may cause high blood pressure to rise even higher at times.

Overdose/Toxicity

Signs and symptoms:
Unlikely to threaten life or cause significant symptoms.

What to do:
For symptoms of overdose:
Discontinue amino acid and consult doctor. Also see *Adverse Reactions or Side Effects* section below.

For accidental overdose (such as child taking entire bottle): Dial 911 (emergency), 0 for operator or call your nearest Poison Control Center.

Adverse Reactions or Side Effects

Reaction or effect	What to do
Lowers blood pressure	Discontinue. Call doctor immediately.
Migraine headaches	Discontinue. Call doctor immediately.
Raises blood pressure	Discontinue. Call doctor immediately.

Interaction with Medicine, Minerals or Vitamins

Interacts with	Combined effect
Antidepressant drugs (containing mono-amine oxidase inhibitors)	Dangerous or life-threatening blood-pressure elevation.
Phenylalanine	Additive effect with tyrosine greatly increases chance of undesirable side effects.

Lab Tests to Detect Deficiency

None are available, except for experimental purposes.

AMINO ACIDS

Food Supplements

The substances discussed in
this section are not minerals,
vitamins or acids. There are
many more supplements
available than those listed in
this book. Many people
continue to debate their value
in human nutrition and health.

Acidophilus (Lactobacillus)

Basic Information

Acidophilus is a bacterium found in yogurt, kefir and other products.

Chemical this supplement contains: enzymes to aid digestion

Known Effects

- Helps maintain normal bacteria balance in lower intestines
- Kills monilia, yeast and fungus on contact

Miscellaneous information:
Acidophilus is made by fermenting milk using *lactobacillus acidophilus* and other bacteria.

Possible Additional Effects

- May lower cholesterol
- May clear up skin problems
- May help prevent vaginal yeast infections in women who take antibiotics or who have diabetes
- May extend life span
- Potential aid for digestion of milk and milk products in people with lactase deficiency
- May enhance immunity
- May reduce symptoms from spastic colon
- May reduce diarrhea related to long-term antibiotic use
- May reduce diarrhea related to chemotherapy or radiation therapy

Warnings and Precautions

Don't take if you:
- Have intestinal problems, except under medical supervision
- Plan to use in vaginal area for yeast infections

Consult your doctor if you:
Take any medicinal drugs or herbs including aspirin, laxatives, cold and cough remedies, antacids, vitamins, minerals, amino acids, supplements, other prescription or nonprescription drugs.

Pregnancy:
Problems in pregnant women taking small or usual amounts have not been proved, but the chance of problems does exist. Don't use unless prescribed by your doctor.

Breastfeeding:
Problems in breastfed infants of lactating mothers taking small or usual amounts have not been proved, but the chance of problems does exist. Don't use unless prescribed by your doctor.

Infants and children:
Treating infants and children under 2 with any supplement is hazardous.

Others:
No problems expected if you are not pregnant and do not take amounts larger than the manufacturer's recommended dosage.

Storage:
- Store in cool, dry place away from direct light, but don't freeze.
- Store safely out of reach of children.
- Don't store in bathroom medicine cabinet. Heat and moisture may change the action of the supplement.

Safe dosage:
- At present no "safe" dosage has been established.
- It is available as a liquid, in capsules or tablets, as a powder or in milk products, such as yogurt or kefir.

Toxicity

Comparative-toxicity rating is not available from standard references.

Adverse Reactions, Side Effects or Overdose Symptoms

None are expected.

Bee Pollen

Basic Information

Bee pollen is the microscopic male seed in flowering plants. It is expensive and provides inadequate, uncertain quantities of nutrients.

Chemicals this supplement contains:
- Amino acids
- Minerals
- Vitamins

Known Effects

None are proven.

Miscellaneous information:
Bee pollen from a local source is preferable as it is more likely to decrease allergy symptoms.

Possible Additional Effects

- May produce antimicrobial (see Glossary) effect
- May renew skin
- May boost immunity
- May decrease allergy symptoms

Warnings and Precautions

Don't take if you:
- Are pregnant, think you may be pregnant or plan pregnancy in the near future.
- Have asthma or allergies to honey or bee stings

Consult your doctor if you:
Take this herb for any medical problem that doesn't improve in 2 weeks (There may be safer, more effective treatments.)

Pregnancy:
Problems in pregnant women taking small or usual amounts have not been proved, but the chance of problems does exist. Don't use unless prescribed by your doctor.

Breastfeeding:
Problems in breastfed infants of lactating mothers taking small or usual amounts have not been proved, but the chance of problems does exist. Don't use unless prescribed by your doctor.

Infants and children:
Treating infants and children under 2 with any supplement is hazardous.

FOOD SUPPLEMENTS

Storage:
- Store in cool, dry place away from direct light, but don't freeze.
- Store safely out of reach of children.
- Don't store in bathroom medicine cabinet. Heat and moisture may change the action of the supplement.

Safe dosage:
- At present no "safe" dosage has been established.
- Bee pollen is available in injectable form and capsules.

Toxicity

Comparative-toxicity rating is not available from standard references.

For symptoms of toxicity: See *Adverse Reactions, Side Effects or Overdose Symptoms* section below.

Adverse Reactions, Side Effects or Overdose Symptoms

Signs and symptoms	What to do
May cause allergic reactions in those sensitive to pollens: Mild allergic response is characterized by itching, pain at injection site and swelling occurring within 24 to 48 hours.	Discontinue. Call doctor immediately.
Life-threatening anaphylaxis may follow injection: Symptoms include immediate severe itching, paleness, low blood pressure, loss of consciousness, coma.	Yell for help. Don't leave victim. Begin CPR (cardio-pulmonary resuscitation), mouth-to-mouth breathing and external cardiac massage. Have someone dial "0" (operator) or 911 (emergency). Don't stop CPR until help arrives.

Bioflavonoids (Vitamin P)

Basic Information

Bioflavonoids are a brightly colored, chemical constituent of the pulp and rind of citrus fruits, green pepper, apricots, cherries, grapes, papaya, tomatoes and broccoli.

There are at least 4,000 compounds found in fruits, vegetables, wine and tea.

For information about specific phyto-chemicals, their food sources and disease prevention, see the *Phytochemicals and Health* chart, pages 184–185.

Chemicals this supplement contains:
- Eriodictyol
- Hesperetin
- Hesperidin
- Nobiletin
- Quercetin
- Rutin
- Sinensetin
- Tangeretin

Known Effects

Treats rare bioflavonoid deficiency characterized by fragile capillaries and unusual bleeding

Miscellaneous information:
- Enough bioflavonoids are present in food to make supplements unnecessary in healthy humans.
- Commercial products such as tablets or capsules often contain vitamin C.

Possible Additional Effects

- Quercetin may help regulate blood-sugar levels in diabetics
- May act as an antioxidant (see Glossary), preventing vitamin C and adrenaline from being oxidized by copper-containing enzymes (see Glossary)
- May increase effectiveness of vitamin C
- May prevent hemorrhoids
- May prevent miscarriages
- May prevent retinal bleeding in people with diabetes and hypertension
- May prevent capillary fragility
- May prevent nosebleed
- May prevent post-partum hemorrhage
- May prevent menstrual disorders
- May prevent blood clotting and platelet clumping
- May prevent easy bruising
- May prevent or treat cataracts
- May lessen symptoms of oral herpes when taken with vitamin C
- May decrease cholesterol levels
- Quercetin may lessen or prevent asthma symptoms

Warnings and Precautions

Don't take if you:
Have a bleeding problem, until studies are done to diagnose the underlying disease.

Consult your doctor if you:
- Self-medicate
- Take any medicinal drugs or herbs including aspirin, laxatives, cold and cough remedies, antacids, vitamins, minerals, amino acids, supplements, other prescription or nonprescription drugs

Pregnancy:
Notify your doctor if you take supplements.

Breastfeeding:
Notify your doctor if you take supplements.

Infants and children:
Treating infants and children under 2 with any supplement is hazardous.

Others:
None are expected if you are beyond childhood and under 45, basically healthy and take supplements for only a short time.

Storage:
- Store in cool, dry place away from direct light, but don't freeze.
- Store safely out of reach of children.
- Don't store in bathroom medicine cabinet. Heat and moisture may change the action of the supplement.

Safe dosage:
- At present no "safe" dosage has been established.
- Bioflavonoids are sold under the brand names Rutin and Hesperiden and are included in numerous vitamin/mineral supplements.

Toxicity

Comparative-toxicity rating is not available from standard references.

Adverse Reactions, Side Effects or Overdose Symptoms

None are expected.

FOOD SUPPLEMENTS

Brewer's Yeast

 Basic Information

Brewer's yeast is nonleavening with a slightly bitter taste. It is an excellent source of B vitamins, protein and minerals.

Chemicals this supplement contains:
- B vitamins
- DNA and RNA (see Glossary)
- Trace mineral, chromium

 Known Effects

- Supplies B vitamins, protein and minerals
- Provides bulk to prevent constipation
- Good source of enzyme-producing vitamins
- Chromium in brewer's yeast helps regulate sugar metabolism

Miscellaneous information:
- Out of the can, the bitter taste of brewer's yeast may be unpleasant. Adding it to foods with a strong taste makes it tolerable.
- Brewer's yeast is a good, inexpensive food supplement for aging adults and growing, developing children.

 Possible Additional Effects

- May reduce risk of high cholesterol in blood
- Possible treatment for contact dermatitis
- May increase energy
- May reduce risk of prostate cancer

 Warnings and Precautions

Don't take if you:
Have intestinal disease.

Consult your doctor if you:
- Have an acute intestinal upset
- Take any medicinal drugs or herbs including aspirin, laxatives, cold and cough remedies, antacids, vitamins, minerals, amino acids, supplements, other prescription or nonprescription drugs
- Have osteoporosis

Pregnancy:
Safe to use in doses of 1 to 2 tablespoons per day.

Breastfeeding:
Safe to use in doses of 1 to 2 tablespoons per day.

Infants and children:
Treating infants and children under 2 with any supplement is hazardous.

Others:
- The quality and quantity of nutrients vary greatly among commercially available products.
- Brewer's yeast is usually nontoxic if you consume 1 tablespoon or less of the powder or equivalent amounts of tablets or flakes.

Storage:
- Store in cool, dry place away from direct light, but don't freeze.
- Store safely out of reach of children.
- Don't store in bathroom medicine cabinet. Heat and moisture may change the action of the supplement.

Safe dosage:
- Brewer's yeast is available in powder, flakes and tablets.
- It can be used in baking, soups, chili and casseroles to increase nutritional content.

Toxicity

Comparative-toxicity rating is not available from standard references.

For symptoms of toxicity: See *Adverse Reactions, Side Effects or Overdose Symptoms* section below.

Adverse Reactions, Side Effects or Overdose Symptoms

Signs and symptoms	What to do
Diarrhea	Discontinue. Call doctor immediately.
Nausea	Discontinue. Call doctor immediately.

Chondroitin Sulfate

Basic Information

This substance is found in the cartilage of most mammals.

Chemicals this supplement contains: complex protein molecules

Known Effects

None are proven.

Miscellaneous information:
Chondroitin sulfate is found in bone, cartilage and connective tissue.

Possible Additional Effects

- May lower cholesterol levels
- May prolong clotting time
- May reduce urine acid levels associated with gout
- Anti-inflammatory effects may reduce osteoarthritis symptoms (generally taken with glucosamine)

Warnings and Precautions

Don't take if you:
- Have bleeding problems
- Are pregnant, think you may be pregnant or plan pregnancy in the near future

Consult your doctor if you take:
- Anticoagulants
- Any medicinal drugs or herbs including aspirin, laxatives, cold and cough remedies, antacids, vitamins, minerals, amino acids, supplements, other prescription or nonprescription drugs

Pregnancy:
Don't use unless prescribed by your doctor.

FOOD SUPPLEMENTS

→

Breastfeeding:
Don't use unless prescribed by your doctor.

Infants and children:
Treating infants and children under 2 with any supplement is hazardous.

Others:
No precautions if you are beyond childhood and under 45, basically healthy and take for only a short time.

Storage:
• Store in cool, dry place away from direct light, but don't freeze.
• Store safely out of reach of children.
• Don't store in bathroom medicine cabinet. Heat and moisture may change the action of the supplement.

Safe dosage:
• At present no "safe" dosage has been established.
• Chondroitin sulfate is available in capsule form.

Toxicity

Comparative-toxicity rating is not available from standard references.

Adverse Reactions, Side Effects or Overdose Symptoms

None are expected.

Coenzyme Q (CoQ) (Ubiquinone)

Basic Information

Coenzyme Q is part of the mitochondria (see Glossary) of cells and is necessary for energy production.

Chemical this supplement contains: coenzyme Q10 (a nutrient) found in

• Beef
• Mackerel
• Peanuts
• Salmon
• Sardines
• Spinach

Known Effects

• Controls flow of oxygen within individual cells
• Increases circulation
• Boosts the immune system

Possible Additional Effects

• May improve heart-muscle metabolism
• Potential treatment for chest pain caused by narrowed coronary arteries (coronary insufficiency)
• May lower blood pressure
• May treat congestive (see Glossary) heart failure by enhancing pumping action of heart
• May be effective in congestive heart failure, ischemic (see Glossary) heart disease

Warnings and Precautions

Don't take if you:
Have heart disease, without consulting your doctor.

Consult your doctor if you:

Take any medicinal drugs or herbs including aspirin, laxatives, cold and cough remedies, antacids, vitamins, minerals, amino acids, supplements, other prescription or nonprescription drugs.

Pregnancy:

Dangers outweigh any benefits. Don't use.

Breastfeeding:

Dangers outweigh any benefits. Don't use.

Infants and children:

Treating infants and children under 2 with any supplement is hazardous.

Others:

No problems are expected if you are not pregnant and do not take amounts larger than the manufacturer's recommended dosage.

Storage:

• Store in cool, dry place away from direct light, but don't freeze.

• Store safely out of reach of children.
• Don't store in bathroom medicine cabinet. Heat and moisture may change the action of the supplement.

Safe dosage:

• 200–300mg, 2 to 3 times per day.
• Oral products are available: Lozenges, chewable tablets and oil-based gelcaps.
• The best forms to use are liquid or oil that contain a small portion of vitamin E to preserve ubiquinone.

 Toxicity

Comparative-toxicity rating is not available from standard references.

 Adverse Reactions, Side Effects or Overdose Symptoms

None are expected.

Conjugated Linoleic Acid (CLA)

 Basic Information

Conjugated linoleic acid is a fatty acid found in corn oil, safflower oil, sunflower oil, canola oil, nuts, seeds, beef and dairy products.

 Known Effects

The following effects have been found in studies conducted on animals, not in humans:

• Reduces body fat
• Inhibits tumor growth
• Boosts immune system

Miscellaneous information:

• CLA is not damaged by cooking or storage.
• CLA is an omega-6 fatty acid.
• The balance between omega-6 and omega-3 fatty acids is important to overall health and disease prevention.
• Linoleic acid is an essential fatty acid that should be included in all diets to prevent a deficiency.
• CLA prevents essential-fatty-acid deficiency due to lack of linoleic acid.

FOOD SUPPLEMENTS

→

Possible
Additional Effects

- May reduce risk of arteriosclerosis
- May reduce cholesterol levels
- May reduce symptoms of psoriasis

 Warnings and
Precautions

Don't take if you:
Are healthy and eat a well-balanced diet.

Consult your doctor if you:
Take anticoagulants.

Pregnancy:
Decide with your doctor if any benefits of CLA justify the risk to your unborn child. Risk is unknown because CLA is not regulated by the FDA.

Breastfeeding:
Breast milk is considered balanced in fatty acids to best meet the infant's needs. Supplements should not be necessary. Consult doctor before taking.

Infants and children:
Treating infants and children under 2 with any supplement is hazardous.

Storage:
- Store in cool, dry place away from direct light, but don't freeze.
- Store safely out of reach of children.
- Don't store in bathroom medicine cabinet. Heat and moisture may change the action of the supplement.

Safe dosage:
CLA, as a product, is marketed as a dietary supplement and is not reviewed by the U.S. Food and Drug Administration (FDA) for effectiveness and safety. The best dosage amounts are unknown. Use with caution.

 Toxicity

Comparative-toxicity rating is not available from standard references.

 Adverse Reactions,
Side Effects or
Overdose Symptoms

None are known.

Creatine

 Basic Information

Creatine is manufactured in the liver and also found in meats.

Chemicals this supplement contains: proteins

 Known Effects

- Promotes weight gain
- Increases muscle strength in athletes
- Increases muscle strength in patients with neuromuscular disease like multiple sclerosis

Miscellaneous information:
- Competitive athletes may benefit from additional amounts of creatine.
- Creatine aids the release of energy in muscles by increasing the production and circulation of adenosine triphosphate (ATP).
- Creatine is not researched carefully as yet for use in humans.

 Possible
Additional Effects

- May improve strength and power

- May enhance performance in activities that require intense short-term effort such as weight-lifting or swimming
- May decrease fatigue

Warnings and Precautions

Don't take if you:
Are allergic to creatine.

Consult your doctor if you:
- Have any chronic health problem
- Are allergic to any medication, food or other substance
- Are considering taking creatine (safety of creatine supplements is currently being investigated by the U.S. Food and Drug Administration)

Pregnancy:
Risk is unknown. Do not use.

Breastfeeding:
Risk is unknown. Do not use.

Infants and children:
Treating infants and children under 2 with any supplement is hazardous.

Others:
- Don't take with any prescription or nonprescription medicine without consulting your doctor or pharmacist.
- Not much is known about the effects of long-term use.

Storage:
- Store in cool, dry place away from direct light, but don't freeze.
- Store safely out of reach of children.
- Don't store in bathroom medicine cabinet. Heat and moisture may change the action of the supplement.

Safe dosage:
- Creatine, as a product, is marketed as a dietary supplement. The U.S. Food and Drug Administration (FDA) recently labeled creatine supplements as unsafe due to deaths in three athletes. It is unknown if creatine or some impurity in the supplement led to the deaths. The best dosage amounts are unknown. Use with caution.
- Creatine is available as chewable tablets, capsules or powder. Follow instructions on the label or consult your doctor or pharmacist. Different brands supply different doses.
- At present no "safe" dosage has been established.

Toxicity

Comparative-toxicity rating is not available from standard references.

For symptoms of toxicity: See *Adverse Reactions, Side Effects or Overdose Symptoms* section below.

Adverse Reactions, Side Effects or Overdose Symptoms

Signs and symptoms	What to do
Gastrointestinal problems	Discontinue. Call doctor when convenient.
Increased blood pressure	Discontinue. Call doctor when convenient.
Muscle cramping	Discontinue. Call doctor when convenient.
Nausea	Discontinue. Call doctor when convenient.

FOOD SUPPLEMENTS

Dehydroepiandrosterone (DHEA)

Basic Information

DHEA is a steroid produced in the human body by the adrenal glands (which sit on top of the kidney).

Known Effects

Improves overall feeling of well-being in some individuals

Miscellaneous information:

- DHEA concentration peaks at about age 20 and then decreases progressively with advancing age. Supplements are sold as an antiaging remedy.
- Although it is not known whether DHEA itself causes hormonal effects, the body breaks DHEA down into two hormones: estrogen and testosterone. Some people's bodies make large amounts of estrogen and testosterone from DHEA, while others make smaller amounts.

Possible Additional Effects

- May treat heart disease
- May improve energy
- May increase strength
- May boost immunity
- May increase muscle
- May decrease fat
- May improve sense of well-being in those with AIDS or multiple sclerosis
- May help reduce symptoms associated with lupus

Warnings and Precautions

Don't take if you:
Are allergic to DHEA.

Consult your doctor if you have:
- Any chronic health problem
- A family history of cancer
- Allergies to any medication, food or other substance

Pregnancy:
Decide with your doctor if any benefits of DHEA justify risk to the unborn child. Risk is unknown because DHEA is not regulated by the FDA.

Breastfeeding:
It is unknown if DHEA passes into milk. Avoid it or discontinue nursing until you finish medicine. Consult doctor for advice on maintaining milk supply.

Infants and children:
Treating infants and children under 2 with any supplement is hazardous.

Others:
- Hormone supplements may not have the same effects on the body as naturally produced hormones have, because the body processes them differently. Higher doses of supplements may result in higher amounts of hormones in the blood than are healthy.
- DHEA is not researched carefully as yet for use in humans. Most research has been performed on animals. Studies are ongoing to find more definite answers about its effect on aging, muscles and the immune system. Studies in men and women have shown an improvement in the feeling of well-being. AIDS patients and those with multiple sclerosis also reported improvement in well-being, but without a change in their disease outcome.
- Researchers are concerned that DHEA supplements may cause high levels of estrogen or testosterone in

some people. The body's own testosterone plays a role in prostate cancer, and high levels of naturally produced estrogen are suspected of increasing breast cancer risk. The effect of DHEA is unknown.
- Don't take with any prescription or nonprescription medicine without consulting your doctor or pharmacist.

Storage:
- Store in cool, dry place away from direct light, but don't freeze.
- Store safely out of reach of children.
- Don't store in bathroom medicine cabinet. Heat and moisture may change the action of the supplement.

Safe dosage:
- DHEA is available in tablet or capsule form: Follow instructions on the label or consult your doctor or pharmacist. Different brands supply different doses. DHEA, as a product, is marketed as a dietary supplement and is not reviewed by the U.S. Food and Drug Administration (FDA) for effectiveness and safety. The best dosage amounts are unknown. Use with caution.

- A lower starting dosage may be recommended for persons over 55 years old until a response is determined.

Toxicity
Comparative-toxicity rating is not available from standard references.

For symptoms of toxicity: See *Adverse Reactions, Side Effects or Overdose Symptoms* section below.

Adverse Reactions, Side Effects or Overdose Symptoms

Signs and symptoms	What to do
Infrequent:	
In women—acne, hair loss, facial hair growth (hirsutism), deepening of voice (the last two may be irreversible)	Discontinue. Call doctor when convenient.

Dessicated Liver

Basic Information
Dessicated liver is a concentrated form of dried liver.

Chemicals this supplement contains:
- Calcium
- Cholesterol
- Copper
- Iron
- Phosphorus
- Vitamins A, B-complex, C, D

Known Effects
Source of vitamins A, B-complex, C, D and iron, calcium, phosphorus, copper

Miscellaneous information:
Do not use. There is a high risk of impurities, especially hepatitis. There is no indication that any organ parts have biological activity after digestion: If you

→

have liver damage or liver problems, eating liver supplements will not fix your liver.

Possible Additional Effects

- May act as an antistress agent
- May cure gum problems
- Possible anemia treatment
- May create red blood cells
- May increase energy

Warnings and Precautions

Don't take if you:
Are pregnant, think you may be pregnant or plan pregnancy in the near future.

Consult your doctor if you:
Take any medicinal drugs or herbs including aspirin, laxatives, cold and cough remedies, antacids, vitamins, minerals, amino acids, supplements, other prescription or nonprescription drugs.

Pregnancy:
Problems in pregnant women taking small or usual amounts have not been proved, but the chance of problems does exist. Don't use unless prescribed by your doctor.

Breastfeeding:
Problems in breastfed infants of lactating mothers taking small or usual amounts have not been proved, but the chance of problems does exist. Don't use unless prescribed by your doctor.

Infants and children:
Treating infants and children under 2 with any supplement is hazardous.

Storage:
- Store in cool, dry place away from direct light, but don't freeze.
- Store safely out of reach of children.
- Don't store in bathroom medicine cabinet. Heat and moisture may change the action of the supplement.

Safe dosage:
- At present no "safe" dosage has been established.
- Dessicated liver is available in tablet or powder form.

Toxicity

Comparative-toxicity rating is not available from standard references.

Adverse Reactions, Side Effects or Overdose Symptoms

None are expected.

Dietary Fiber

Basic Information

Cell walls of plants are made of fiber that give a plant structure and stability. Fiber cannot be broken down by enzymes in the digestive tract, so fiber passes through without being absorbed.

Chemicals this supplement contains: structured and nonstructured substances in plant carbohydrate (starches)

Soluble Food Sources	Insoluble Food Sources
Apples	Brown rice
Barley	Legumes
Citrus fruits	Nuts
Cooked dried beans	Raw vegetables
Oats/oat bran/oatmeal	Root vegetables
Strawberries	Seeds
	Wheat bran
	Whole-grain breads and cereals

Known Effects

- Absorbs many times its weight in water, causing bulkier stools and lessening chance of constipation
- Helps control blood-sugar level in diabetics
- Helps reduce cholesterol and triglycerides in blood
- Soluble fiber found in oats is particularly beneficial for lowering cholesterol

Miscellaneous information:

- The best sources of dietary fiber include fresh fruits, vegetables, nuts, seeds, whole-grain products and potatoes.
- Increase in diet gradually over several weeks to avoid gastro-intestinal distress.

Possible Additional Effects

- May reduce risk of heart disease
- May reduce risk of colon and rectum cancer
- May reduce risk of diverticulitis
- May reduce risk of hemorrhoids
- May reduce risk of obesity
- Wheat, bran fiber may reduce risk of breast cancer

Warnings and Precautions

Don't take if you:
Have Crohn's disease.

Consult your doctor if you:
Are pregnant, think you may be pregnant or plan pregnancy in the near future.

Pregnancy:
Problems in pregnant women taking small or usual amounts have not been proved, but the chance of problems does exist. Don't use unless prescribed by your doctor.

Breastfeeding:
Problems in breastfed infants of lactating mothers taking small or usual amounts have not been proved, but the chance of problems does exist. Don't use unless prescribed by your doctor.

Infants and children:
Treating infants and children under 2 with any supplement is hazardous.

Others:
- Intake of excessive amounts of fiber may decrease absorption of minerals, especially calcium, iron and zinc.
- Take fiber supplements separately from vitamin and mineral supplements.

Storage:
- Store in cool, dry place away from direct light, but don't freeze.
- Store safely out of reach of children.
- Don't store in bathroom medicine cabinet. Heat and moisture may change the action of the supplement.

Safe dosage:
- Most experts feel that increasing fiber is healthful.
- Recommended intake to reduce risk of heart disease and cancer and promote blood-glucose control is 25–30 grams per day. →

FOOD SUPPLEMENTS

- Fiber is available commercially in capsules, tablets, chewable tablets, oral suspension and flakes or wafers.

Toxicity

Comparative-toxicity rating is not available from standard references.

For symptoms of toxicity: See *Adverse Reactions, Side Effects or Overdose Symptoms* section below.

Adverse Reactions, Side Effects or Overdose Symptoms

Signs and symptoms	What to do
Bloating of abdomen	Discontinue. Call doctor when convenient.
Excess flatulence	Discontinue. Call doctor when convenient.
Obstruction of large intestine (rare, but more likely if there is pre-existing inflammatory disease): Symptoms of obstruction are tender, distended abdomen; abdominal pain; fever; no bowel movements.	Discontinue. Call doctor immediately.

Gamma Linolenic Acid (GLA)

Basic Information

Gamma linolenic acid is found in a supplement called *evening primrose oil.*

Chemicals found in this supplement: fatty acids found in

- Evening primrose (a plant)
- Fish
- Human mother's milk
- Spirulina (blue-green algae)

Known Effects

- Astringent
- Anti-inflammatory
- Reduces liver damage

- Anticoagulant properties, which make it useful in the prevention of heart attacks caused by thrombosis
- Helps people suffering from atopic eczema or eczema due to allergy
- Source of essential fatty acids

Miscellaneous information:

- Deficiency can cause eczema.
- Those whose fat and oil intake is greatly restricted may require supplements.
- Evening primrose grows wild. A long spike of yellow flowers opens at night. Oil can be expressed from the tiny seeds of the flower.

Possible Additional Effects

- Used in external preparations to treat skin eruptions, such as psoriasis
- May reduce inflammation associated with arthritis

Warnings and Precautions

Don't take if you are:
- Healthy and eat a well-balanced diet
- On anticoagulant therapy—may increase bleeding time
- Taking other medicines such as phenothiazines, tricyclic antidepressants or anticonvulsants

Consult your doctor if you:
Have any illness.

Pregnancy:
GLA appears to be safe. Consult your doctor before taking.

Breastfeeding:
GLA appears to be safe. Consult your doctor before taking.

Infants and children:
Treating infants and children under 2 with any supplement is hazardous.

Others:
- Gamma linolenic acid, working with enzymes, becomes part of some prostaglandins. Prostaglandins sometimes limit inflammatory reactions in the body and sometimes cause inflammatory reactions. Taking evening primrose oil may cause unpredictable, harmful effects.
- Patients with schizophrenia should avoid taking gamma linolenic acid.

- Discontinue at least 2 weeks prior to any surgery.
- Taking with vitamin E may prevent oxidation of the oil.

Storage:
- Store in cool, dry place away from direct light, but don't freeze.
- Store safely out of reach of children.
- Don't store in bathroom medicine cabinet. Heat and moisture may change the action of the supplement.

Safe dosage:
- GLA is available in capsule form: Swallow whole with a full glass of liquid. Don't chew or crush. Take with or 1 to 1-1/2 hours after meals unless otherwise directed by your doctor.
- At present, no "safe" dosage has been established.

Toxicity

Unlikely to threaten life or cause significant symptoms.

For symptoms of toxicity: See *Adverse Reactions, Side Effects or Overdose Symptoms* section below.

Adverse Reactions, Side Effects or Overdose Symptoms

Signs and symptoms	What to do
Headache, indigestion, nausea	Discontinue. Call doctor when convenient.

FOOD SUPPLEMENTS

Inositol

Basic Information

Inositol is also called *myoinositol*.

- Breast milk
- Calf liver
- Cantaloupe
- Citrus fruit (except lemons)
- Dried beans
- Garbanzo beans (chickpeas)
- Lentils
- Milk
- Nuts
- Oats
- Pork
- Rice
- Veal
- Wheat germ
- Whole-grain products

Known Effects

- Plays a role similar to choline in helping move fats out of liver
- Functions in nerve transmission
- Forms an important part of phospholipids, which are compounds manufactured in our bodies

Miscellaneous information:

- Individuals under medical supervision for sleep or anxiety disorders may benefit from supplements.
- Newborns benefit from inositol through breast milk.

Possible Additional Effects

- May protect against peripheral neuropathy associated with diabetes (Some studies have shown promise for this use, but definitive, well-controlled studies have not been done.)
- May function as mild antianxiety agent
- May help control blood-cholesterol level
- Potential treatment for constipation with its stimulating effect on muscular action of alimentary canal
- May improve sleep
- Under study for anxiety disorders and Alzheimer's disease

Warnings and Precautions

Don't take if you:
Are healthy.

Consult your doctor if you:

- Have diabetes with peripheral neuropathy: pain, numbness, tingling, alternating feelings of cold and hot in feet and hands—medical supervision is necessary
- Have a sleep or anxiety disorder

Pregnancy:
Don't take.

Breastfeeding:
Don't take.

Infants and children:
Treating infants and children under 2 with any supplement is hazardous

Others:
Excretion may increase with lithium treatment.

Storage:

- Store in cool, dry place away from direct light, but don't freeze.
- Store safely out of reach of children.
- Don't store in bathroom medicine cabinet. Heat and moisture may change the action of the supplement.

Safe dosage:

- At present, no "safe" dosage has been established.

- Inositol is available in capsule form: Swallow whole with a full glass of liquid. Don't chew or crush. Take with or 1 to 1-1/2 hours after meals unless otherwise directed by your doctor.

 Toxicity

Unlikely to threaten life or cause significant symptoms.

 Adverse Reactions, Side Effects or Overdose Symptoms

None are expected.

Jojoba (Goatnut)

 Basic Information

Biological name: *Simmondsia chinensis.*

Chemicals this supplement contains: amino acids

 Known Effects

Acts as soothing ingredient in many shampoos, toothpastes, pre-electric-shave conditioners, aftershave preparations, skin lotion, makeup remover

Miscellaneous information:
- Jojoba is unique among plants because its seeds contain a liquid wax oil.
- The plant grows in Arizona and is used as a medicinal herb among Southern Arizona Indians.
- Jojoba is used in perfume.

 Possible Additional Effects

- May reduce joint pain associated with rheumatoid arthritis
- May relieve swelling
- May promote healing
- Potential dry skin treatment

 Warnings and Precautions

Don't take if you:
No problems are expected if you are an adult and not pregnant or breastfeeding and do not take amounts larger than the manufacturer's recommended dosage.

Consult your doctor if you:
- Are pregnant, think you may be pregnant or plan pregnancy in the near future
- Take any medicinal drugs or herbs including aspirin, laxatives, cold and cough remedies, antacids, vitamins, minerals, amino acids, supplements, other prescription or nonprescription drugs

FOOD SUPPLEMENTS

→

Pregnancy:

Problems in pregnant women taking small or usual amounts have not been proved, but the chance of problems does exist. Don't use unless prescribed by your doctor.

Breastfeeding:

Problems in breastfed infants of lactating mothers taking small or usual amounts have not been proved, but the chance of problems does exist. Don't use unless prescribed by your doctor.

Infants and children:

Treating infants and children under 2 with any supplement is hazardous.

Others:

No beneficial effects when taken by mouth have been proved.

Storage:

• Store in cool, dry place away from direct light, but don't freeze.

• Store safely out of reach of children.
• Don't store in bathroom medicine cabinet. Heat and moisture may change the action of the supplement.

Safe dosage:

At present no "safe" dosage has been established.

Toxicity

Comparative-toxicity rating is not available from standard references.

Adverse Reactions, Side Effects or Overdose Symptoms

None are expected.

L-Carnitine

Basic Information

L-carnitine is synthesized in the body from the amino acids *lysine* and *methionine*. It is found naturally in avocados, breast milk, dairy products, red meats (especially lamb and beef) and tempeh (fermented soybean product).

Known Effects

• Promotes normal growth and development

• Essential for infants, especially premature infants
• Transports long-chain fatty acids into mitochondria, which are the metabolic furnaces of cells (particularly heart and kidney cells), where they may be oxidized to yield energy
• Synthesized in human kidney and liver from the essential amino acids lysine and methionine, plus vitamin B-6, vitamin C and iron

Miscellaneous information:

• Because carnitine requires essential amino acids to be synthesized by the body, anyone with deficient protein or amino acids in their diet may require supplements.

• People with recent severe burns or injuries, hypothyroidism and vegan vegetarians may also require supplements. Consult your doctor.

Possible Additional Effects

• Possible treatment for (and maybe prevention of) some forms of cardiovascular disease
• May protect against muscle disease
• May help build muscle
• May protect against liver disease
• May protect against diabetes
• May protect against kidney disease
• Potential diet aid
• May make low-calorie diets easier to tolerate by reducing feelings of hunger and weakness
• May increase energy and activity in people with congestive heart disease (see Glossary)

Warnings and Precautions

Don't take if you are:
• Allergic to any food protein, such as eggs, milk, wheat
• At risk of poor nutrition for any reason
• Pregnant, think you may be pregnant or plan pregnancy in the near future

Consult your doctor if you:
Have any liver or kidney problems.

Pregnancy:
Problems in pregnant women taking small or usual amounts have not been proved, but the chance of problems does exist. Don't use unless prescribed by your doctor.

Breastfeeding:
Problems in breastfed infants of lactating mothers taking small or usual amounts have not been proved, but the chance of problems does exist. Don't use unless prescribed by your doctor.

Infants and children:
Treating infants and children under 2 with any supplement is hazardous.

Others:
• Deficiency may cause muscle fatigue, cramps or low blood-sugar levels.
• AZT may reduce carnitine levels.

Storage:
• Store in cool, dry place away from direct light, but don't freeze.
• Store safely out of reach of children.
• Don't store in bathroom medicine cabinet. Heat and moisture may change the action of the supplement.

Safe dosage:
• At present no "safe" dosage has been established.
• Available as tablets: Swallow whole with a full glass of liquid. Don't chew or crush. Take with or 1 to 1-1/2 hours after meals unless otherwise directed by your doctor. Avoid DL-carnitine tablets; they may be toxic.
• Also available as acetyl L-carnitine.

Toxicity

Comparative-toxicity rating is not available from standard references.

For symptoms of toxicity: See *Adverse Reactions, Side Effects or Overdose Symptoms* section below.

FOOD SUPPLEMENTS

→

Adverse Reactions, Side Effects or Overdose Symptoms

Signs and symptoms	What to do
Muscle weakness	Discontinue. Consult doctor.
Symptoms of myasthenia (progressive weakness of certain muscle groups without evidence of atrophy or wasting) have been reported in kidney patients being maintained for prolonged periods on hemodialysis and supplemental DL-carnitine.	Don't take supplements without doctor's prescription and supervision.

Lecithin

Basic Information

Lecithin is also called *phosphatidyl-choline.*

Lecithin is found in all animal and plant products.

Chemicals this supplement contains:

• Choline
• Fatty acids
• Glycerin
• Phosphorus

Known Effects

• Protects against damage to cells by oxidation
• Major source of the chemical nutrient choline—choline's benefits are also lecithin's benefits (see Choline)

Miscellaneous information:

• Lecithin must be present for choline synthesis in the human body.
• It is found in chemicals that aid passage of many nutrients from the bloodstream into cells.
• It is used as a thickener in several foods, including mayonnaise, margarine and ice cream.
• People taking niacin or nicotinic acid for treatment of high-serum cholesterol and triglycerides may need lecithin or choline supplements.

Possible Additional Effects

- May protect against cardiovascular disease
- May treat liver damage caused by alcoholism
- May lower cholesterol level

Warnings and Precautions

Don't take if you:
Are healthy and eat a well-balanced diet.

Consult your doctor if you:
Plan to treat Alzheimer's disease with lecithin/choline.

Pregnancy:
Supplements are unnecessary.

Breastfeeding:
Supplements are unnecessary.

Infants and children:
Treating infants and children under 2 with any supplement is hazardous.

Others:
- Excess lecithin may increase phosphorus levels unless the diet is adequate in calcium.
- It may cause inaccurate results in a lecithin/sphingomyelin lab test as part of an examination of amniotic fluid.
- Nicotinic acid (nicotinamide, vitamin B-3) decreases lecithin effectiveness.

Storage:
- Store in cool, dry place away from direct light, but don't freeze.
- Store safely out of reach of children.
- Don't store in bathroom medicine cabinet. Heat and moisture may change the action of the supplement.

Safe dosage:
- Don't take more than 1 gram per day.
- Lecithin is available as tablets: Swallow whole with a full glass of liquid. Don't chew or crush. Take with or 1 to 1-1/2 hours after meals unless otherwise directed by your doctor.
- Lecithin is also available in liquid form: Dilute in at least 1/2 glass of water or other liquid. Take with or 1 to 1-1/2 hours after meals unless otherwise directed by your doctor.

Toxicity

Comparative-toxicity rating is not available from standard references.

For symptoms of toxicity: See *Adverse Reactions, Side Effects or Overdose Symptoms* section below.

Adverse Reactions, Side Effects or Overdose Symptoms

Signs and symptoms	What to do
Dizziness	Discontinue. Call doctor immediately.
Fishy body odor	Discontinue. Call doctor when convenient.
Nausea or vomiting	Discontinue. Call doctor immediately.

FOOD SUPPLEMENTS

Melatonin

Basic Information

Melatonin is a hormone produced in the body by the pineal gland and secreted at night. In most people, melatonin levels are highest during the normal hours of sleep. The levels increase rapidly in the late evening, peaking after midnight and decreasing toward morning.

Known Effects

- Fatigue
- Helps alleviate sleep disturbances
- Helps cure insomnia and restless leg syndrome

Miscellaneous information:
Melatonin is not yet researched carefully for use in humans.

Possible Additional Effects

- May slow aging
- May fight disease
- May enhance sex life
- May diminish the effects of jet lag

Warnings and Precautions

Don't take if you:
Are allergic to melatonin.

Consult your doctor if you have:
- Any chronic health problem
- Allergies to any medication, food or other substance
- High blood pressure (hypertension) or cardiovascular disease (Some studies in animals suggest melatonin may constrict blood vessels, a condition that could be dangerous for people with these conditions.)

Pregnancy:
Decide with your doctor if the benefits of melatonin justify the risk to your unborn child. The risk is unknown because melatonin is not regulated by the FDA.

Breastfeeding:
It is unknown if melatonin passes into milk. Consult your doctor before taking.

Infants and children:
Treating infants and children under 2 with any supplement is hazardous.

Others:
- Don't take with any prescription or nonprescription medicine without consulting your doctor or pharmacist.
- Drivers, pilots or individuals involved in hazardous work should not work while using melatonin until it has been determined how it affects them.
- Alcohol and tobacco disrupt the nighttime melatonin effect. Avoid.

Storage:
- Store in cool, dry place away from direct light, but don't freeze.
- Store safely out of reach of children.
- Don't store in bathroom medicine cabinet. Heat and moisture may change the action of the supplement.

Safe dosage:
- Melatonin, as a product, is marketed as a dietary supplement and is not reviewed by the U.S. Food and Drug Administration (FDA) for effectiveness and safety. The best

dosage amounts are unknown. Use with caution.

- Hormone supplements may not have the same effects on the body as naturally produced hormones have, because the body processes them differently. Higher doses of supplements may result in higher amounts of hormones in the blood than are healthy.
- Melatonin is available in tablet or capsule form: Follow instructions on the label or consult your doctor or pharmacist. Different brands supply different doses.
- At present "safe" dosage information is unknown.
- A lower starting dosage is often recommended for people over 55 years old until a response is determined.

Toxicity

Comparative-toxicity rating is not available from standard references.

For symptoms of toxicity: See *Adverse Reactions, Side Effects or Overdose Symptoms* section below.

Adverse Reactions, Side Effects or Overdose Symptoms

Signs and symptoms	What to do
Drowsiness, confusion, headache or grogginess may occur the following morning.	Reduce dosage or discontinue. Call doctor when convenient.

Omega-3 Fatty Acids (Fish Oils)

Basic Information

Omega-3 fatty acids are a dietary supplement available in capsules or oil. These acids come from cold-water fish, particularly cod, tuna, salmon, halibut, shark and mackerel.

Chemicals this supplement contains:
- Docosahexaenoic acid (DHA)
- Eicosapentaenoic acid (EPA)

Known Effects

- Greenland Eskimos who eat foods high in omega-3 fatty acids have very low serum triglycerides and total cholesterol. They have high high-density-lipoprotein (HDL) cholesterol. This cholesterol is known to protect against deposits of plaque, which can occlude (see Glossary) critical blood vessels and cause heart attacks, strokes and other major health problems. Coastal Japanese people have similar diets and similar findings. Increasing omega-3 by supplementation may raise blood cholesterol.
- Omega-3 acids protect against coronary artery disease.
- They also protect against arteriosclerosis.

Miscellaneous information:

Increasing "oily" fish in the diet is preferable to taking omega-3 fatty-acid supplements.

→

FOOD SUPPLEMENTS

Possible Additional Effects

- Potential anti-inflammatory for arthritis
- May protect against strokes
- May improve immune response
- May impede blood clotting
- May increase tendency toward anemia in menstruating women
- May reduce reclosure of arteries after angioplasty

Warnings and Precautions

Don't take if you:
- Are pregnant, think you may be pregnant or plan pregnancy in the near future
- Are diabetic, as supplements are high in fat
- Have a blood-clotting problem (omega-3 acids may impede clotting)

Consult your doctor if you:

Take any medicinal drugs or herbs including aspirin, laxatives, cold and cough remedies, antacids, vitamins, minerals, amino acids, supplements, other prescription or nonprescription drugs.

Pregnancy:

Problems in pregnant women taking small or usual amounts have not been proved, but the chance of problems does exist. Don't use unless prescribed by your doctor.

Breastfeeding:

Problems in breastfed infants of lactating mothers taking small or usual amounts have not been proved, but the chance of problems does exist. Don't use unless prescribed by your doctor.

Infants and children:

Treating infants and children under 2 with any supplement is hazardous.

Others:
- This fat becomes rancid easily and quickly.
- No one knows how much is beneficial and nontoxic.
- Omega-3 causes fishy breath odor, greasy stools, belching and abdominal distension.
- It reduces blood-clotting capability and could cause excessive bleeding in an accident.
- People are generally advised to discontinue 3 to 4 weeks prior to elective surgery.
- Heat kills essential fatty acids, so they should not be processed or cooked.

Storage:
- Store in cool, dry place away from direct light, but don't freeze.
- Store safely out of reach of children.
- Don't store in bathroom medicine cabinet. Heat and moisture may change the action of the supplement.

Safe dosage:

At present no "safe" dosage has been established.

Toxicity

Comparative-toxicity rating is not available from standard references.

For symptoms of toxicity: See *Adverse Reactions, Side Effects or Overdose Symptoms* section below.

Adverse Reactions, Side Effects or Overdose Symptoms

Signs and symptoms	What to do
Large amounts may lead to bleeding problems, diminished immunity, predisposition to some malignancies.	Discontinue. Call doctor immediately.

Para-Aminobenzoic Acid (PABA)

 ## Basic Information

Para-aminobenzoic acid is made by intestinal bacteria and can be found in the following foods: bran, brown rice, kidney, liver, molasses, sunflower seeds, wheat germ, whole-grain products and yogurt.

Chemicals this supplement contains: enzymes, to aid the breakdown and synthesis of protein

 ## Known Effects

- Shields skin from ultraviolet radiation damage when used as a topical sunscreen
- Treats vitiligo, a condition characterized by discoloration or depigmentation of some areas of the skin
- Increases effectiveness of folic acid, vitamin-B complex and vitamin C

Miscellaneous information:

PABA stimulates intestinal bacteria, enabling them to produce folic acid, which aids in the production of pantothenic acid.

 ## Possible Additional Effects

- May rejuvenate skin
- May treat arthritis
- May treat constipation
- May treat gastrointestinal disorders
- May treat nervousness and irritability

 ## Warnings and Precautions

Don't take if you:

Take any sulfonamide or antibiotic internally because PABA prevents them from exerting their full effect.

Consult your doctor if you:

Are pregnant, think you may be pregnant or plan pregnancy in the near future.

Pregnancy:
- Don't take internally. Risks outweigh the benefits.
- No problems are expected if you use PABA topically.

Breastfeeding:
- Don't take internally. Risks outweigh the benefits.
- No problems are expected if you use PABA topically.

Infants and children:

Treating infants and children under 2 with any supplement is hazardous.

Others:
- Decreases effectiveness of antibiotics
- Decreases effectiveness of sulfonamides ("sulfa drugs")

Storage:
- Store in cool, dry place away from direct light, but don't freeze.
- Store safely out of reach of children.
- Don't store in bathroom medicine cabinet. Heat and moisture may change the action of the supplement.

Safe dosage:
- At present no "safe" dosage has been established.

FOOD SUPPLEMENTS

- PABA is a constituent of many multivitamin/mineral preparations: Don't take oral supplements without your doctor's supervision.
- PABA is a constituent of many topical sunscreen products.

 Toxicity

PABA is stored in the tissues. In continued high doses, it may prove toxic to the liver. Symptoms of toxicity are nausea and vomiting.

For symptoms of toxicity:
Discontinue supplement and consult doctor. Also see *Adverse Reactions, Side Effects or Overdose Symptoms* section below.

 Adverse Reactions, Side Effects or Overdose Symptoms

Signs and symptoms	What to do
Diarrhea	Discontinue. Call doctor immediately.
Fever	Discontinue. Call doctor immediately.
Liver disease, evidenced by abnormal liver-function tests, jaundice (yellow skin and eyes), vomiting	Discontinue. Call doctor immediately.
Nausea or vomiting	Discontinue. Call doctor immediately.
Skin rash	Discontinue. Call doctor immediately.

Pregnenolone

 Basic Information

Pregnenolone is used by the body to make steroids. It increases estrogen and testosterone levels in the body.

 Known Effects

None are proven.

Miscellaneous information:
- Pregnenolone is not researched carefully as yet for use in humans. Most research has been performed on animals. Studies are ongoing to find more definite answers about its effect on aging and memory.
- It is a precursor (see Glossary) of DHEA (see DHEA).

 Possible Additional Effects

- May improve memory
- May slow the aging process
- May aid in treating spinal cord injury when used with anti-inflammatory agents
- May reduce inflammation associated with arthritis

 Warnings and Precautions

Don't take if you:
- Are allergic to pregnenolone
- Have a hormone-dependent cancer or cancer history in your family

Consult your doctor if you have:
- Any chronic health problem
- Allergies to any medication, food or other substance

Pregnancy:
Decide with your doctor if the benefits of pregnenolone justify the risk to your unborn child. Risk is unknown because pregnenolone is not regulated by the FDA.

Breastfeeding:
It is unknown if pregnenolone passes into milk. Consult your doctor before taking.

Infants and children:
Treating infants and children under 2 with any supplement is hazardous.

Others:
Don't take with any prescription or nonprescription medicine without consulting your doctor or pharmacist.

Storage:
- Store in cool, dry place away from direct light, but don't freeze.
- Store safely out of reach of children.
- Don't store in bathroom medicine cabinet. Heat and moisture may change the action of the supplement.

Safe dosage:
- Pregnenonlone, as a product, is marketed as a dietary supplement and is not reviewed by the U.S. Food and Drug Administration (FDA) for effectiveness and safety. The best dosage amounts are unknown. Use with caution.

- Hormone supplements may not have the same effects on the body as naturally produced hormones have, because the body processes them differently. Higher doses of supplements may result in higher amounts of hormones in the blood than are healthy.
- A lower starting dosage may be recommended for persons over 55 years old until a response is determined.
- Pregnenolone is available in capsule form: Follow instructions on the label or consult your doctor or pharmacist. Different brands supply different doses.

 Toxicity

Comparative-toxicity rating is not available from standard references.

For symptoms of toxicity: See *Adverse Reactions, Side Effects or Overdose Symptoms* section below.

 Adverse Reactions, Side Effects or Overdose Symptoms

Signs and symptoms	What to do
Infrequent:	
In women—facial hair growth (hirsutism) **In men—breast enlargement**	Discontinue. Call doctor when convenient.

Royal Jelly

Basic Information

Royal jelly is a milky-white, gelatinous substance secreted by the salivary glands of worker bees to stimulate growth and development of queen bees.

Chemicals this supplement contains: pantothenic acid (part of B-complex vitamins)

Known Effects

None are proven.

Miscellaneous information:
This substance must be given by injection.

Possible Additional Effects

- May extend life span
- May treat bone and joint disorders, such as rheumatoid arthritis
- May protect against leukemia
- May contain antibiotic properties
- May treat bronchial asthma
- May treat insomnia
- May treat liver and kidney disease

Warnings and Precautions

Don't take if you:
Are pregnant, think you may be pregnant or plan pregnancy in the near future.

Consult your doctor if you:
Take any medicinal drugs or herbs including aspirin, laxatives, cold and cough remedies, antacids, vitamins, minerals, amino acids, supplements, other prescription or nonprescription drugs.

Pregnancy:
Dangers outweigh any benefits. Don't use.

Breastfeeding:
Dangers outweigh any benefits. Don't use.

Infants and children:
Treating infants and children under 2 with any supplement is hazardous.

Others:
Dangers outweigh any benefits. Don't use.

Storage:
- Store safely out of reach of children.
- Keep refrigerated in a tightly sealed container.

Safe dosage:
At present no "safe" dosage has been established.

Toxicity

Comparative-toxicity rating is not available from standard references.

For symptoms of toxicity: See *Adverse Reactions, Side Effects or Overdose Symptoms* section below.

Adverse Reactions, Side Effects or Overdose Symptoms

Signs and symptoms	What to do
Life-threatening anaphylaxis may follow injections: Symptoms include immediate severe itching, paleness, low blood pressure, loss of consciousness, coma.	Yell for help. Don't leave victim. Begin CPR (cardio-pulmonary resuscitation), mouth-to-mouth breathing and external cardiac massage. Have someone dial "0" (operator) or 911 (emergency). Don't stop CPR until help arrives.

Shark Cartilage

Basic Information

Shark cartilage is made from the powdered cartilage of shark.

Chemicals this supplement contains:
- Amino acids (some)
- Calcium
- Mucopolysaccharides
- Phosphorus
- Protein

Known Effects

Mucopolysaccharides found in this cartilage inhibit the growth of new blood vessels (cellular angiogenesis).

Miscellaneous information:
Some doctors question the effectiveness of taking oral shark-cartilage supplements. They feel that the supplement's active ingredient may be destroyed during digestion, not allowing it to enter the bloodstream.

Additionally, there is no objective evidence to suggest it protects against cancer.

Possible Additional Effects

- May boost immune system
- May decrease joint swelling and stiffness due to anti-inflammatory properties
- Because of angiogenesis-inhibition properties, it may be effective in the treatment of certain eye disorders that occur because of inappropriate growth of new blood vessels, as well as arthritis, psoriasis, bowel inflammation, scleroderma

FOOD SUPPLEMENTS

→

Warnings and Precautions

Don't take if you:
- Have recently undergone surgery
- Have had a heart attack
- Are still growing

Consult your doctor if you:
Take any prescription or nonprescription medicine.

Pregnancy:
Decide with your doctor if any benefits of shark cartilage justify the risk to your unborn child. Risk is unknown because shark cartilage is not regulated by the FDA.

Breastfeeding:
It is unknown if shark cartilage passes into milk. Consult your doctor before taking.

Infants and children:
Treating infants and children under 2 with any supplement is hazardous.

Storage:
- Store in cool, dry place away from direct light, but don't freeze.
- Store safely out of reach of children.
- Don't store in bathroom medicine cabinet. Heat and moisture may change the action of the supplement.

Safe dosage:
- Shark cartilage, as a product, is marketed as a dietary supplement and is not reviewed by the U.S. Food and Drug Administration (FDA) for effectiveness and safety. The best dosage amounts are unknown. Use with caution.
- Shark cartilage is available in powder or capsule form: It is important to get a supplement that is 100% pure shark cartilage to get the maximum effect. The color should be white.

Toxicity

Comparative-toxicity rating is not available from standard references.

Adverse Reactions, Side Effects or Overdose Symptoms

None are known.

Spirulina (Blue-Green Algae)

Basic Information

Biological names: *Spirulina maxima, Spirulina platensis.*

Chemicals this supplement contains:

- B-complex vitamins
- Beta-carotene
- Gamma-linolenic acid
- Iron
- Protein

Known Effects

None are proven.

Miscellaneous information:
- Spirulina is expensive and tastes terrible.
- It is a blue-green microalgae that grows wild on the surface of brackish, alkaline lakes in the tropics.

• Spirulina is cultivated commercially in several places, including Mexico, Thailand, Japan and Southern California.

Possible Additional Effects

• Possible energy booster
• May protect immune system
• May lower cholesterol
• May decrease appetite
• May be beneficial for individuals with hypoglycemia

Warnings and Precautions

Don't take if you:

Are pregnant, think you may be pregnant or plan pregnancy in the near future.

Consult your doctor if you:

Take any medicinal drugs or herbs including aspirin, laxatives, cold and cough remedies, antacids, vitamins, minerals, amino acids, supplements, other prescription or nonprescription drugs.

Pregnancy:

Don't use unless prescribed by your doctor.

Breastfeeding:

Don't use unless prescribed by your doctor.

Infants and children:

Treating infants and children under 2 with any supplement is hazardous.

Others:

No problems are expected if you are not pregnant and do not take amounts larger than a reputable manufacturer recommends on the package.

Storage:

• Keep in cool, dry place away from direct light, but don't freeze.
• Store safely out of reach of children.
• Don't store in bathroom medicine cabinet. Heat and moisture may change the action of the supplement.

Safe dosage:

• At present no "safe" dosage has been established.
• Spirulina is available in powder and tablet form. Follow manufacturer's instructions or consult your doctor.

Toxicity

Comparative-toxicity rating is not available from standard references.

For symptoms of toxicity: See *Adverse Reactions, Side Effects or Overdose Symptoms* section below.

Adverse Reactions, Side Effects or Overdose Symptoms

Signs and symptoms	What to do
Diarrhea	Discontinue. Call doctor immediately.
Nausea	Discontinue. Call doctor immediately.
Vomiting	Discontinue. Call doctor immediately.

FOOD SUPPLEMENTS

Superoxide Dismutase

Basic Information

Superoxide dismutase is an enzyme associated with copper, zinc and manganese.

Chemical this supplement contains: enzyme that participates in utilization of copper, zinc and manganese by body cells

Known Effects

- Neutralizes the free radical (see Glossary) superoxide
- Protects against free radicals

Possible Additional Effects

- May reduce oxidative cell damage associated with cancer, cancer therapies
- May have antioxidant (see Glossary) properties (injectable forms only)

Warnings and Precautions

Don't take if you:
Have any medical problems.

Consult your doctor if you:
Take any medicinal drugs or herbs including aspirin, laxatives, cold and cough remedies, antacids, vitamins, minerals, amino acids, supplements, other prescription or nonprescription drugs.

Pregnancy:
Don't use without medical supervision.

Breastfeeding:
Don't use without medical supervision.

Infants and children:
Treating infants and children under 2 with any supplement is hazardous.

Others:
- Available oral forms are worthless.
- Injectable forms may cause anaphylaxis.

Storage:
- Store in cool, dry place away from direct light, but don't freeze.
- Store safely out of reach of children.
- Don't store in bathroom medicine cabinet. Heat and moisture may change the action of the supplement.

Safe dosage:
- At present no "safe" dosage has been established.
- Oral superoxide dismutase is destroyed in the intestines before being absorbed, so oral forms are worthless unless pills are enteric-coated to allow absorption into the small intestines.
- It is available in injectable forms, but these should be used only under close medical supervision.

Toxicity

Comparative-toxicity rating is not available from standard references.

For symptoms of toxicity: *See Adverse Reactions, Side Effects or Overdose Symptoms section below.*

Adverse Reactions, Side Effects or Overdose Symptoms

Signs and symptoms	What to do
Life-threatening anaphylaxis may follow injections: Symptoms include immediate severe itching, paleness, low blood pressure, loss of consciousness, coma.	Yell for help. Don't leave victim. Begin CPR (cardio-pulmonary resuscitation), mouth-to-mouth breathing and external cardiac massage. Have someone dial "0" (operator) or 911 (emergency). Don't stop CPR until help arrives.

Wheat Germ

Basic Information

Wheat germ is the embryo of the wheat grain, located at the lower end. It is derived from both root and shoot.

Chemicals this supplement contains:

- Calcium
- Copper
- Magnesium
- Manganese
- Most B vitamins
- Phosphorus
- Vitamin E (one of the richest natural sources)

Known Effects

Excellent nutritional source of chemicals listed above

Possible Additional Effects

- May reduce symptoms of muscular dystrophy
- May improve physical stamina and performance

Warnings and Precautions

Don't take if you:

No problems are expected if you are not pregnant and do not take amounts larger than manufacturer's recommended dosage.

Consult your doctor if you:

- Are pregnant, think you may be pregnant or plan pregnancy in the near future
- Take any medicinal drugs or herbs including aspirin, laxatives, cold and cough remedies, antacids, vitamins, minerals, amino acids, supplements, other prescription or nonprescription drugs

Pregnancy:

Problems in pregnant women taking small or usual amounts have not been proved, but the chance of problems does exist. Don't use unless prescribed by your doctor.

➜

FOOD SUPPLEMENTS

Breastfeeding:
Problems in breastfed infants of lactating mothers taking small or usual amounts have not been proved, but the chance of problems does exist. Don't use unless prescribed by your doctor.

Infants and children:
Treating infants and children under 2 with any supplement is hazardous.

Others:
No problems are expected if you are beyond childhood and under 45, basically healthy and take for only a short time.

Storage:
• Keep cool and dry, but don't freeze.
• Store safely out of reach of children.
• Wheat germ goes rancid quickly—keep refrigerated.

Safe dosage:
• At present no "safe" dosage has been established.
• Wheat germ is available in food and as flakes to mix with other foods. It is also available as oil, which should be kept tightly covered and refrigerated.

 Toxicity

Comparative-toxicity rating is not available from standard references.

 Adverse Reactions, Side Effects or Overdose Symptoms

None are expected.

Wheat Grass (Barley Grass, Plant Sprouts)

 Basic Information

These products are derived from roots and leaves.

Chemicals this supplement contains:

• B vitamins
• Chlorophyll
• Select phytochemicals
• Superoxide dismutase

 Known Effects

None are proven.

 Possible Additional Effects

• May protect against cancer
• May function as an antioxidant

 Warnings and Precautions

Don't take if you:
Are pregnant, think you may be pregnant or plan pregnancy in the near future.

Consult your doctor if you take:
• This supplement for any medical problem that doesn't improve in 2 weeks (There may be safer, more effective treatments.)

• Any medicinal drugs or herbs including aspirin, laxatives, cold and cough remedies, antacids, vitamins, minerals, amino acids, supplements, other prescription or nonprescription drugs.

Pregnancy:

Problems in pregnant women taking small or usual amounts have not been proved, but the chance of problems does exist. Don't use unless prescribed by your doctor.

Breastfeeding:

Problems in breastfed infants of lactating mothers taking small or usual amounts have not been proved, but the chance of problems does exist. Don't use unless prescribed by your doctor.

Infants and children:

Treating infants and children under 2 with any supplement is hazardous.

Others:

No problems are expected if you are not pregnant and do not take amounts larger than the manufacturer's recommended dosage.

Storage:

• Store in cool, dry place away from direct light, but don't freeze.
• Store safely out of reach of children.
• Don't store in bathroom medicine cabinet. Heat and moisture may change the action of the supplement.

Safe dosage:

At present no "safe" dosage has been established.

Toxicity

Comparative-toxicity rating is not available from standard references.

Adverse Reactions, Side Effects or Overdose Symptoms

None are expected.

Optimal Daily Intake Information

Vitamin or Mineral	Daily Value (DV)	Recommended Dietary Allowances	Dietary Reference Intakes	Tolerable Upper Intake	Probable Optimal Intake for Disease
A	5,000IU	Men 1,000mcg Women 800mcg			5,000IU
Asorbic Acid		60mg	60mg		250–500mg
B-12	6mcg	2mcg	2.4mcg		2.4–10mcg
Calcium	1,000mg	800–1,200mg	1,000–1,200mg	2,500mg	1,200–1,500mg
Choline			Men 550mg Women 425mg	3,500mg	375–550mg
Chromium					50–150mcg
Copper	2mg				2–3mg
D	400IU	5–10mcg	5–10mcg	50mcg	400–600IU
E	30IU	Men 10mg Women 8mg			400IU
Fluoride			Men 4mg Women 3mg	10mg	2–10mg
Folic Acid/ Folate	400mcg	Men 200mcg Women 180mcg	400mcg	1,000mcg (synthetic folic acid)	400–800mcg
Iodine	150mcg	150mcg			150mcg
Iron	18mg	Men 10mg Women 15mg			Supplement only if a deficiency exists
Magnesium	400mg	Men 350mg Women 280mg	Men 400–420mg Women 310–320mg	350mg (from pharmacological source only)	500–1,000mg

About This Chart:

The amounts listed in this chart are recommended for healthy adults.

Daily Value (DV) is a standard set forth by the Food and Drug Administration (FDA). It combines Reference Daily Intakes (RDI) and Daily Recommended Values (DRV). DRVs were developed to cover nutrients that are not included in RDIs. The term DV is used in food labeling. You should use it as a reference for determining how much of your nutrient needs are being met through the consumption of a specific food.

Recommended Dietary Allowances (RDA), Dietary Reference Intakes (DRI) and Tolerable Upper Intake Level (UL) are determined by the Food and Nutrition Board of the Institute of Medicine, National Academy of Sciences.

RDAs determine the minimum amount of a nutrient needed to prevent deficiency.

Vitamin or Mineral	Daily Value (DV)	Recommended Dietary Allowances	Dietary Reference Intakes	Tolerable Upper Intake	Probable Optimal Intake for Disease
Manganese					2–5mg
Molybdenum					75–250mcg
Niacin (B-3)	20mg	Men 15–19mg Women 13–15mg	Men 16mg Women 14mg	35mg	15–35mg
Pantothenic Acid (B-5)	10mg		5mg		5–20mg
Phosphorus	1,000mg	800–1,200mg	700mg	4,000mg	1,200–1,500mg
Phytonadione		Men 70–80mcg Women 60–65mcg			Supplement not required in healthy diet
Potassium	3,500mg				4,000mg
Pyridoxine (B-6)	2mg	Men 2mg Women 1.6mg	1.3–1.7mg	100 mg	1.5–50mg
Riboflavin (B-2)	1.7mg	Men 1.4–1.7mg Women 1.2–1.3mg	Men 1.3mg Women 1.1mg		1.3–50mg
Selenium		Men 70mcg Women 55mcg			100mcg
Sodium	2,400mg				2,400mg
Thiamine (B-1)	1.5mg	Men 1.2–1.5mg Women 1–1.1mg	Men 1.2mg Women 1.1mg		1.2–50mg
Zinc	15mg	Men 15mg Women 12mg			15–25mg

Reprinted with permission from *Dietary Reference Intakes.* Copyright 1998 by the National Academy of Sciences. Courtesy of the National Academy Press, Washington, D.C.

DRIs will expand upon RDAs by focusing on optimal health and the use of nutrients in promoting long-term health.

UL determines the maximum nutrient intake without risk of side effects, when the scientific evidence is available.

DRI guidelines are being announced in phases. The project is expected to be complete by 2001.

Sources:

DV information was taken from the U.S. Food and Drug Administration website: http://www.fda.gov

RDA, DRI and UL information was taken from the Food and Nutrition Board, Institute of Medicine, National Academy of Sciences—Dietary Reference Intakes: recommended levels for individual intake.

OPTIMAL DAILY INTAKE

Phytochemicals and Health

Phytochemicals are chemicals found in or derived from plants.

Phytochemicals and Disease Prevention		
Phytochemical	**Food source(s)**	**Clinical significance**
Alpha linolenic acid	flaxseed, soy, walnuts	reduces inflammation, lowers blood cholesterol, may protect against breast cancer, enhances immunity
Beta-carotene	green and yellow fruits and vegetables	reduces risk of cataracts, coronary artery disease, lung and breast cancers; enhances immunity (elderly)
Capsaicin	chili peppers	reduces risk for colon, gastric and rectal cancer; inhibits tumor promotion
Carotenoid, lycopene	tomato sauce, catsup, red grapefruit, guava, dried apricots, watermelon, fresh tomatoes	antioxidant, reduces risk of prostate cancer, may reduce cardiovascular disease
Curcumin	turmeric, curry, cumin	may lower cholesterol, reduces risk of skin cancer
Cynarin	artichokes	decreases cholesterol levels
Ellagic acid	wine, grapes, currants, nuts (pecans), berries (strawberries, blackberries, raspberries), seeds	reduces cancer risk, inhibits carcinogen binding to DNA, reduces LDL cholesterol while increasing HDL cholesterol
Flavonols, polyphenols: catechin (theaflavins, thearubigins), theogallin, EGCG	green and black tea, berries	reduces risk of gastric cancer, antioxidant, increases immune function, decreases cholesterol production, protects against chemically induced cancers and skin cancer, may protect against esophageal cancer, antitumor promoter, inhibits nitrosamine formation, inhibits phase I and enhances phase II enzyme activity
Genistein	soybeans	reduces risk of hormone-dependent cancers; alters hormone levels; inhibits angiogenesis; promotes cell differentiation; reduces cholesterol levels; reduces thrombi formation, osteoporosis, menopausal symptoms
Indoles	cabbage, broccoli, Brussels sprouts, spinach, watercress, cauliflower, turnips, kohlrabi, kale, rutabaga, horseradish, mustard greens	reduces risk of hormone-related cancers, may "inactivate" estrogen, increases glutathione-S-transferase activity, inhibits growth of transformed cells

Phytochemical	Food source(s)	Clinical significance
Isothiocyanates, sulforaphane	cabbage, cauliflower, broccoli and broccoli sprouts, Brussels sprouts, mustard greens, horseradish, radishes	reduces risk of tobacco-induced tumors, inhibits tobacco-related carcinogens from damaging DNA, induces phase II enzymes, inhibits cP450 activation of carcinogens
Lignans	high fiber foods, especially seeds	reduces cancer risk (colon), reduces blood glucose and cholesterol
Monterpene, limonene	citrus (peel, membrane), mint, caraway, thyme, coriander	antioxidant, reduces cancer risk (skin, breast), inhibits p21ras (G protein), suppresses HMG-CoA, induces apoptosis, reduces cholesterol production, reduces premenstrual symptoms
Organosulfur compounds, allylic acid	garlic, onion, watercress, cruciferous vegetables, leeks	decreases lipid peroxidation; reduces risk of gastric, colon and lung cancers; inhibits tumor promotion by inhibiting DNA adduct formation; induces phase II enzymes; antithrombotic; reduces cholesterol; reduces blood pressure; antimicrobial
Phenolic acid	cruciferous vegetables, eggplant, peppers, tomatoes, celery, parsley, soy, licorice root, flaxseed, citrus, whole grains, berries	inhibits cancer by inhibiting nitrosamine formation, reduces risk for lung and skin cancers
Polyacetylene	parsley, carrots, celery	decreases risk of tobacco-induced tumors, alters prostaglandin formation
Quercetin	pear skin, apple skin, bell pepper, kohlrabi, tomato leaves, onion, wine, grape juice	flavonoid, anticancer, antioxidant, associated with reduced coronary heart disease, decreases platelet aggregation

PHYTOCHEMICALS AND HEALTH

Glossary

abortifacient. Induces abortions (miscarriages).

absorption. Process by which nutrients are absorbed through the lining of the intestinal tract into capillaries and into the bloodstream. Nutrients must be absorbed to affect the body.

acute. Short, relatively severe. Usually referred to in connection with an illness. Opposite of acute is *chronic*.

addiction. Psychological or physiological dependence on a drug. With true addictions, severe symptoms appear when the addicted person stops taking the drug on which he or she is dependent.

adrenal gland. Gland located immediately adjacent to the kidney that produces epinephrine (adrenaline) and several steroid hormones, including cortisone and hydro-cortisone.

adulterant. Substance that makes another substance impure when the two are mixed together.

allergen. Capable of producing an allergic response.

allergy. Excessive sensitivity to a substance.

alpha linolenic acid. An essential fatty acid important for healing and maintaining good health.

alumina. Another term for aluminum oxide or hydrated aluminum oxide.

amenorrhea. Absence of menstruation.

amino acid. Chemical building blocks that help produce proteins in the body.

anabolic. Building up of tissues in the body, or constructive metabolism.

analog. Employing measurement along scales rather than by numerical counting.

anaphylaxis. Severe allergic response to a substance. Symptoms include wheezing, itching, nasal congestion, hives, immediate intense burning of hands and feet, collapse with severe drop in blood pressure, loss of consciousness and cardiac arrest. Symptoms of anaphylaxis appear within a few seconds or minutes after exposure to the substance causing reaction—this can be medication or herbs taken by injection, by mouth, vaginally, rectally, through a breathing apparatus or applied to skin. Anaphylaxis is an uncommon occurrence, but when it occurs, it is a *severe medical emergency!* Without appropriate immediate treatment, it can cause death. Yell for help. Don't leave victim. Begin CPR (cardiopulmonary resuscitation), mouth-to-mouth breathing and external cardiac massage. Have someone dial "0" or 911. Don't stop CPR until help arrives.

anemia. Too few healthy red blood cells in the bloodstream or too little hemoglobin in the red blood cells. Anemia is usually caused by excessive blood loss, such as excessive bleeding or menstruation, increased blood destruction, such as hemolytic anemia or leukemia, or decreased blood production, such as iron-deficiency anemia.

anemia, pernicious. Anemia caused by vitamin-B-12 deficiency. Symptoms include easy fatigue, weakness, lemon-colored skin, numbness and tingling of hands and feet, and symptoms of degeneration of the central nervous system, such as irritability, emotional problems, personality changes and paralysis of extremities.

anesthetic. Used to abolish pain.

angina (angina pectoris). Chest pain, with sensation of impending death. Pain may radiate into jaw, ear lobes, between shoulder blades or down shoulder and arm on either side, most frequently the left side. Pain is caused by a temporary reduction in the amount of oxygen to the heart muscle through narrowed, diseased coronary arteries.

antacid. Neutralizes acid. In medical terms, the neutralized acid is located in the stomach, esophagus or first part of the duodenum.

antagonist. A drug that blocks or reverses the effect of another drug.

antibacterial. Destroys bacteria (germs) or suppresses their growth or reproduction.

antibiotic. Inhibits growth of germs or kills germs. When it inhibits growth, it is called *bacteriostatic*. When it kills germs, it is called *bacteriocidal*.

anticholinergic. Reduces nerve impulses through the part of the autonomic nervous system called *parasympathetic*.

anticoagulant. Delays or stops blood clotting.

antiemetic. Prevents or stops nausea and vomiting.

antihelmintic. Destroys intestinal worms.

antihistamine. Reduces *histamine*.

antihypertensive. Reduces blood pressure.

antimicrobial. Destroys or inhibits growth of microorganisms.

antimitotic. Inhibits or prevents cell division.

antineoplastic. Inhibits or prevents growth of neoplasms (cancers).

antioxidant. Prevents or delays the process of *oxidation*. Antioxidant substances include superoxide dismutase, selenium, vitamins C and E and zinc.

antipyretic. Reduces fevers.

antiseptic. Prevents or retards growth of germs.

antispasmodic. Relieves spasm in skeletal or smooth muscle.

apertive. Stimulates the appetite.

artery. Blood vessel that carries blood away from the heart.

asthma. Disease with recurrent attacks of breathing difficulty characterized by wheezing. It is caused by spasms of the bronchial tubes, which can be caused by many factors including adverse reactions to drugs, vitamins, minerals or medicinal herbs.

astringent. Shrinks tissues and prevents secretion of fluids.

bacteria. Microscopic germs. Some bacteria contribute to health; others cause disease.

bioavailability. The degree to which a drug becomes available to the target tissue after administration.

blepharitis. Inflammation of the eyelid.

blood sugar (blood glucose). Necessary element in blood to sustain life. The blood level of glucose is determined by insulin, a hormone secreted by the pancreas. When the pancreas no longer satisfies this function, the disease *diabetes mellitus* results.

bronchitis. Inflammation of the breathing tubes.

carcinogen. Chemical or substance that can cause cancer.

cardiac. Pertaining to the heart.

cardiac arrhythmias. Abnormal heart rate or rhythm.

cardiomyopathy. Chronic disorder of the heart muscle of unknown association.

carminative. Aids in expelling gas from the intestinal tract.

cathartic. Very strong laxative that produces explosive, watery bowel movements.

cell. Unit of protoplasm, the essential living matter of all plants and animals.

central nervous system. Brain and spinal cord and their nerve endings.

central-nervous-system depressant. Causes changes in the body, including changes in consciousness, lethargy, loss of judgment or coma.

GLOSSARY

chronic. Disease of long standing. Opposite of *acute.*

coenzyme. Heat-stable molecule that must be loosely associated with an *enzyme* for the enzyme to perform its function.

cofactor. Element with which another must unite to function.

colic. Abdominal pain that recurs in a pattern every few seconds or minutes.

collagen. Gelatinous protein used to make body tissues.

congestive. Excess accumulation of blood. Congestive heart failure is the result of blood congregating in lungs, liver, kidney and other parts to cause shortness of breath, swelling of ankles, sleep disturbances, rapid heartbeat and easy fatigue.

conjunctivitis. Inflammation of the outer membrane of the eye.

constriction. Tightness or pressure.

contraceptive. Prevents pregnancy.

contraindication. Inadvisability of using a substance that may cause harm under specific circumstances. For example, high-caloric intake in someone who is overweight is contraindicated.

convulsion. Violent, uncontrollable contraction of the voluntary muscles.

corticosteroid (adrenocorticosteroid). Hormones produced by the body or manufactured synthetically.

cystitis. Inflammation of the bladder.

delirium. Temporary mental disturbance accompanied by hallucinations, agitation, incoherence.

demineralization. Excessive elimination of mineral or inorganic salts.

dermatitis. Skin inflammation or irritation.

diaphoretic. Increases perspiration.

diuretic. Increases urine flow. Most diuretics force kidneys to excrete more than the usual amount of sodium. Sodium forces more water and urine to be excreted.

DNA (deoxyribonucleic acid). Complex protein chemical in genes that determines the type of life form into which a cell will develop.

dosage. The amount of medicine to be taken for a specific problem. Dosages may be listed as liquids (ml or milliliters, cc or cubic centimeters, teaspoons, tablespoons), dry weight (kg or kilograms, mg or milligrams, g or grams) or by biological assay (retinol units, international units).

duodenum. First 12 inches of small intestine.

dysentery. Disorder with inflammation of the intestines, especially the colon, accompanied by pain, a feeling of urgent need to have bowel movements, and frequent stools containing blood or mucus.

dysmenorrhea. Painful or difficult menstruation.

dyspepsia. Digestion impairment causing uncomfortable feeling of indigestion.

eczema. Noncontagious disease of skin characterized by redness, itching, scaling and lesions with discharge. Frequently becomes encrusted. Eczema primarily affects young children. The underlying cause is usually an allergy to many things, including foods, wool, skin lotions. The disorder may begin in month-old babies. It usually subsides by age 3 but may flare again at age 10 to 12 and last through puberty.

electrolyte. Chemical substance with an available electron in its atomic structure that can transmit electrical impulses when dissolved in fluids.

emetic. Causes vomiting.

emmenagogue. Triggers onset of menstrual period.

emphysema. Lung disease characterized by loss of elasticity of muscles surrounding air sacs. Lungs cannot supply adequate oxygen to body cells for normal function.

endometriosis. Medical condition in which uterine tissue is found outside the uterus. Symptoms include pain, abnormal menstruation, infertility.

enzyme. Protein chemical that accelerates a chemical reaction in the body without being consumed in the process.

epilepsy. Symptom or disease characterized by episodes of brain disturbance that cause convulsions and loss of consciousness.

estrogens. Female sex hormones that must be present for secondary sexual characteristics of the female to develop. Estrogens serve many functions in the body, including preparation of the uterus to receive a fertilized egg.

eupeptic. Promotes optimum digestion.

expectorant. Decreases thickness and increases fluidity of mucus in the lungs and bronchial tubes.

extremity. Arm, hand, leg, foot.

fat soluble. Dissolves in fat.

fatty acids. Nutritional substances found in nature that are fats or lipids. These include triglycerides, cholesterol, fatty acids and prostaglandins. Fatty acids include stearic, palmitic, linoleic, linolenic, eicosapentaenoic (EPA), docosahexaenoic acid (DHA). Other lipids of nutritional importance include lecithin, choline, gamma linolenic acid and inositol.

flatulence. Swelling of the stomach or other parts of the intestinal tract with air or other gases.

flavonoids. A category of powerful antioxidants.

free radicals. Highly reactive molecules with an unpaired free electron that combines with any other molecule that accepts it. Free radicals are usually toxic oxygen molecules that damage cell membranes and fat molecules. To protect against possible damage from free radicals, the body has several defenses. The most important appear at present to be *antioxidant* substances.

G6PD. Deficiency of glucose-6-phosphate, a chemical necessary for glucose metabolism. Some people have inherited deficiencies of this substance and have added risks when taking some drugs.

GABA (gamma-aminobutyric acid). An amino acid that functions as a neurotransmitter in the *central nervous system.*

gastritis. Inflammation of stomach lining.

gastroenteritis. Inflammation of stomach and intestines characterized by pain, nausea and diarrhea.

gastrointestinal. Pertaining to stomach, small intestine, large intestine, colon, rectum and sometimes the liver, pancreas and gallbladder.

generic. Relating to or descriptive of an entire group or class.

genistein. A component of soybeans thought to be an anticarcinogen.

genitourinary. Relating to the genital and urinary organs and functions.

gingivitis. Inflammation of the gums surrounding teeth.

gland. Cells that manufacture and excrete materials not required for their own metabolic needs.

glossitis. Inflammation of the tongue.

gluten. Mixture of plant proteins occurring in grains, chiefly corn and wheat. People who are sensitive to gluten develop gastrointestinal symptoms that can be controlled only by eating a gluten-free diet.

griping. Intestinal cramps.

hallucinogen. Produces hallucinations —apparent sights, sounds or other sensual experiences that do not actually exist.

HDL (high density lipoprotein). "Good cholesterol" that scavenges excess cholesterol from the bloodstream and carries it to the liver for excretion.

heart block. An electrical disturbance in the controlling system of the heartbeat. Heart block can cause unconsciousness and in its worst form can lead to cardiac arrest.

hematuria. Blood in the urine.

hemoglobin. Pigment necessary for red blood cells to transport oxygen. Iron is a necessary component of hemoglobin.

hemolysis. Breaking a membranous covering or destroying red blood cells.

hemorrhage. Extensive bleeding.

hemostatic. Prevents bleeding and promotes clotting of blood.

hepatitis. Inflammation of liver cells, usually accompanied by *jaundice.*

histamine. Chemical in the body tissues that constricts the smooth muscle surrounding bronchial tubes, dilates small blood vessels, allows leakage of fluid to form itching skin and hives and increases secretion of acid in stomach.

hives. Elevated patches on skin usually caused by an allergic reaction accompanied by a release of *histamine* into the body tissues. Patches are red or pale and itch intensely.

hormone. Chemical substance produced by endocrine glands—thymus, pituitary, thyroid, parathyroid, adrenal, ovaries, testicles, pancreas—that regulates many body functions to maintain homeostasis (a steady state).

hypercalcemia. Abnormally high level of calcium in the blood.

hypercholesterolemia. Excess cholesterol in the blood.

hyperplasia. An unusual increase in the elements composing a part (such as cells composing tissue).

hypertension. High blood pressure.

hypocalcemia. Abnormally low level of calcium in the blood.

hypoglycemia. Abnormally low blood sugar.

impotence. Inability of a male to achieve and maintain an erection of the penis to allow satisfying sexual intercourse.

insomnia. Inability to sleep.

interaction. Change in body's response to one substance when another is taken. Interactions may increase the response, decrease the response, cause toxicity or completely change the response expected from either substance. Interactions may occur between drugs and drugs, drugs and vitamins, drugs and herbs, drugs and foods, vitamins and vitamins, minerals and minerals, vitamins and foods, minerals and foods, vitamins and herbs, herbs and herbs, and so forth.

international units. Measurement of biological activity. In the case of vitamin E, for example, 1 international unit (IU) equals 1 milligram (mg). International units are measured differently for different substances.

ischemia. Localized tissue anemia caused by obstructed blood flow in the arteries.

I.U. or IU. *International units.*

jaundice. Symptom of liver damage, bile obstruction or excessive red-blood-cell destruction. Jaundice is characterized by yellowing of the whites of the eyes, yellow skin, dark urine and light stool.

kidney stones. Small, solid stones made from calcium, cysteine, cholesterol and other chemicals in the bloodstream. They are produced in the kidneys.

lactagogue. Increases the flow of breast milk in a woman.

lactase. *Enzyme* that helps body convert lactose to glucose and galactose.

lactase deficiency. Lack of adequate supply of the enzyme *lactase*. People with lactase deficiency have difficulty digesting milk and milk products.

larvacide. Kills larvae.

laxative. Stimulates bowel movements.

LDH (lactic dehydrogenase). A blood test to measure liver function and to detect damage to the heart muscle.

LDL (low density lipoprotein). "Bad cholesterol" protein that contains large amounts of fats and triglycerides.

libido. Sex drive.

lipid. Fat or fatty substance.

lymph glands. Glands located in the lymph vessels of the body that trap foreign material, including infectious material, and protect the bloodstream from becoming infected.

magnesia. Another term for magnesium hydroxide.

malabsorption. Poor absorption of nutrients from the intestinal tract into the bloodstream.

mcg. Abbreviation for microgram, which is 1/1,000,000th (1/1-millionth) of a gram or 1/1,000th of a milligram.

megadose. Very large dose. In terms of Recommended Dietary Allowance (RDA), anything 10 or more times the RDA is a megadose. Nutritionists urge no one take megadoses of *any* substance because these doses may be toxic, cause an imbalance of other nutrients, cause damage to an unborn child and do not provide benefits beyond rational doses.

menopause. End of menstruation in the female caused by decreased production of female hormones. Symptoms include hot flashes, irritability, vaginal dryness, changes in the skin and bones.

metabolism. Chemical and physical processes in the maintenance of life.

mg. Abbreviation for milligram, which is 1/1,000th of a gram.

migraine. Periodic headaches caused by constriction of arteries in the skull. Symptoms include visual disturbances, nausea, vomiting, light sensitivity and severe pain.

milk sickness. Intolerance to milk and milk products due to a deficiency of an enzyme called *lactase.*

mitochondria. Components of cells, found outside the nucleus, that produce energy for the cell and are rich in fats, proteins and *enzymes.*

mitogen. Causes nucleus of cell to divide; leads to a new cell.

mucilage. Gelatinous substance that contains proteins and polysaccharides.

narcotic. Depresses the central nervous system, reduces pain and causes drowsiness and euphoria. Narcotics are addictive substances.

neuropathy. Group of symptoms caused by abnormalities in sensory or motor nerves. Symptoms include tingling and numbness in hands or feet, followed by gradually progressive muscular weakness.

neurotransmitter. A substance that transmits nerve impulses across a synapse.

occlusion. Obstruction.

osteoporosis. Softening of bones.

oxidation. Combining a substance with oxygen.

oxidation-reduction. A chemical reaction that involves the transfer of an electron from one molecule or atom to another.

oxygenation. Saturation of a substance (particularly blood) with oxygen.

parasympathetic. Division of the autonomic nervous system. Parasympathetic nerves control functions of digestion, heart and lung activity, constriction of eye pupils and many other normal functions of the body.

Parkinson's disease. Disease of the central nervous system characterized by a fixed, emotionless expression of the face, slower-than-normal muscle movements, tremor (particularly when attempting to reach or hold objects), weakness, changed gait and a forward-leaning posture.

paronychia. Fingernail-bed infection.

pellagra. Disease caused by a deficiency of niacin (vitamin B-3). Symptoms include diarrhea, skin inflammation and dementia (brain disturbance).

peristalsis. Wave of contractions of the intestinal tract.

pernicious anemia. See *Anemia, pernicious.*

pharyngitis. Throat inflammation.

phenylketonuria. Inherited disease caused by lack of an *enzyme* necessary for converting phenylalanine into a form the body can use. Accumulation of too much phenylalanine can cause poor mental and physical development in a newborn. Most states require a test at birth to detect the disease. When detected early and treated, phenylketonuria symptoms can be prevented by dietary control.

phosphates. Salts of phosphoric acid. Important part of the body system that controls acid-base balance. Other chemicals involved in acid-base balance include sodium, potassium, bicarbonate and proteins.

photosensitization. Process by which a substance or organism becomes sensitive to light.

photosensitizing pigment. Pigment that makes a substance sensitive to light.

phytochemical. Any one of many substances present in fruits and vegetables that have various health-promoting properties.

platelet aggregation. A collective of individual blood platelets.

GLOSSARY

potassium. Element in body tissue that plays a critical role in electrolyte and fluid balance in the body.

prostate. Gland in the male that surrounds the neck of the bladder and urethra. In older men, it may become infected (prostatitis), obstructed (prostatic hypertrophy), cause urinary difficulties or become cancerous.

psoriasis. Chronic, recurrent skin disease characterized by patches of flaking skin with discoloration.

psychosis. Mental disorder characterized by deranged personality, loss of contact with reality, delusions and hallucinations.

purgative. Powerful laxative usually leading to explosive, watery diarrhea.

purine base. A crystalline base that is the parent of uric-acid compounds. Also a constituent of *DNA* and *RNA*.

purine foods. Foods metabolized into uric acid; these include anchovies, brains, liver, sweetbreads, sardines, meat extracts, oysters, lobster and other shellfish.

pyrimidine base. An organic base. Also a constituent of *DNA* and *RNA*.

quercetin. A pharmacologically active *flavonoid* that inhibits the synthesis of *enzymes* necessary for the release of histamines.

RDA (Recommended Dietary Allowance). Recommendations based on data derived from different population groups and ages. The quoted RDA figures represent the *average* amount of a particular nutrient needed per day to maintain good health in the average healthy person. Data for these recommendations have been collected and analyzed by the Food and Nutrition Board of the National Research Council. These figures are a reference point for comparison. It is only within the framework of statistical probability that RDA can be used legitimately and meaningfully. The Food and Nutrition Board is currently researching a new classification: Dietary Reference Intakes (DRIs), which will include and go beyond RDAs.

renal. Pertaining to the kidneys.

resin. Complex chemicals, usually hard, transparent or translucent, that frequently cause adverse effects in the body.

retina. Inner covering of the eyeball on which images form to be perceived in the brain via the optic nerve.

rickets. Bone disease caused by vitamin-D deficiency. Bones become bent and distorted during infancy or childhood if there is insufficient vitamin D for normal growth and development.

RNA (ribonucleic acid). Complex protein chemical in genes that determines the type of life form into which a cell will develop.

sedative. Reduces excitement or anxiety.

sensory neuropathy. See *neuropathy.*

SGOT. Abbreviation for *serum glutamic oxaloacetic transaminase,* a blood test to measure liver function or detect damage to the heart muscle.

spasmolytic. Decreases spasm of smooth or skeletal (striated) muscle.

steroidal chemicals. Group of chemicals with same properties as steroids. Steroids are fat-soluble compounds with carbon and acid components. They are found in nature in the form of hormones and bile acids, and in plants as naturally occurring drugs, such as digitalis.

stimulant. Stimulates; temporarily arouses or accelerates physiological activity of an organ or organ system.

stomachic. Promotes increased contraction of stomach muscles.

stomatitis. Inflammation of the mouth.

stroke. Sudden, severe attack that results in brain damage. Usually sudden paralysis or speech difficulty results from injury to the brain or spinal cord by a blood clot, hemorrhage or occlusion of blood supply to the brain from a narrowed or blocked artery.

tenesmus. Urgent feeling of having to have a bowel movement or to urinate.

thrombophlebitis. Inflammation of a vein, usually caused by a blood clot. If the clot becomes detached and travels to the lung, the condition is called thromboembolism.

toxicity. Poisonous reaction that impairs body functions or damages cells.

toxin. Poison in dead or live organism.

tranquilizer. Calms a person without clouding mental function.

tremor. Involuntary trembling.

tyramine. Chemical component of the body. In normal quantities, without interference from other chemicals, tyramine helps sustain normal blood pressure. In the presence of some drugs—monoamine oxidase inhibitors and some rauwolfia compounds—tyramine levels can rise and cause toxic or fatal levels in the blood.

urethra. Hollow tube through which urine is transported from the bladder to outside the body. In men, semen is also transported through the urethra from the testicles.

uterus. Hollow, muscular organ in the female in which an embryo develops into a fetus. Menstruation occurs when the lining sloughs periodically.

vein. Vessel that returns blood to the heart.

virus. Infectious organism that reproduces in the cells of an infected host.

water soluble. Dissolves in water.

wax. High-molecular-weight hydrocarbons; they are insoluble in water.

yeast. Single-cell organism that can cause infection of the skin, mouth, vagina, rectum and other parts of the gastrointestinal system. The terms *yeast fungus* and *monilia* are used interchangeably.

Metric Chart

The following units of measurement and weight are commonly used in establishing doses of minerals, supplements and vitamins.

Unit	Abbreviation	Volume	Approximate U.S. Equivalent
Cubic centimeter	cc	0.000001 cubic meter	0.061 cubic inch
Liter	l	1 liter	1.057 quarts
Deciliter	dl	0.10 liter	0.21 quart
Centiliter	cl	0.01 liter	0.338 fluid ounce
Milliliter	ml	0.001 liter	0.27 fluid dram
Kilogram	kg	1,000 grams	2.2046 pounds
Gram	g or gm	1 gram	0.035 ounce
Milligram	mg	0.001 gram	0.015 grain
Microgram	mcg	0.000001 gram	0.0000154 grain

METRIC CHART

Bibliography

American Dietetic Association. *Handbook of Clinical Dietetics.* New Haven, Conn.: Yale University Press, 1981.

American Medical Association. *Drug Evaluations.* 6th ed. Chicago: American Medical Association, 1986.

Balch, James F., M.D., and Phyllis A. Balch, C.N.C. *Prescription for Nutritional Healing.* 2d ed. Garden City Park, N.Y.: Avery Publishing Group, 1997.

Benowicz, Robert J. *Vitamins and You.* New York: Grosset & Dunlap, 1979.

Butler, Kurt, and Lynn Rayner. *The Best Medicine: The Complete Health and Preventive Medicine Handbook.* San Francisco: Harper & Row, 1985.

Clayman, Charles B., M.D., ed. *American Medical Association Encyclopedia of Medicine.* New York: Random House, 1989.

The Complete Book of Vitamins. Emmaus, Pa: Rodale Press, 1984.

Eades, Mary Dan, M.D. *The Doctor's Complete Guide to Vitamins and Minerals.* New York: Dell, 1994.

Edmunds, Marilyn W., ed. *Nursing Drug Reference: A Practitioner's Guide.* Bowie, Md.: Brady Communications Company, 1985.

Eisenhauer, Laurel A. *The Nurse's 1984-85 Guide to Drug Therapy: Drug Profiles for Patient Care.* Englewood Cliffs, N.J.: Prentice-Hall, 1984.

Fischer, William L. *Miracle Healing Power Through Nature's Pharmacy.* Canfield, Ohio: Fischer Publishing Corporation, 1986.

Garrison, Robert, Jr., and Elizabeth Somer. *Nutrition Desk Reference.* New Canaan, Conn.: Keats Publishing, 1985.

Hendler, Sheldon Saul. *The Complete Guide to Anti-Aging Nutrients.* New York: Simon & Schuster, 1985.

Herbert, Victor. *Nutrition Cultism: Facts and Fictions.* Philadelphia: George F. Stickley Company, 1981.

Holford, Patrick. *Vitamin Vitality.* New York: Bantam Books, 1986.

Kirschmann, John D. *Nutrition Almanac.* 2d ed. New York: McGraw-Hill, 1984.

Lasswell, Anita B., et. al. *Nutrition for Family and Primary Care Practitioners.* Philadelphia: George F. Stickley Company, 1986.

Lee, William H. *Kelp, Dulse and Other Sea Supplements.* New Canaan, Conn.: Keats Publishing, 1983.

Lieberman, Shari, Ph.D., and Nancy Bruning. *The Real Vitamin & Mineral Book.* 2d ed. Garden City Park, N.Y.: Avery Publishing Group, 1997.

Marshall, Charles W. *Vitamins and Minerals: Help or Harm?* Philadelphia: George F. Stickley Company, 1983.

McDonald, Arline, Ph.D., R.D., Annette Natow, Ph.D., R.D., JoAnn Heslin, M.A., R.D., and Susan Male Smith, M.A., R.D. *Complete Book of Vitamins & Minerals.* Lincolnwood, Ill.: Publications International, Ltd., 1996.

Merriam-Webster's Collegiate Dictionary. 10th ed. Springfield, Mass.: Merriam-Webster, Inc., 1997.

Mervyn, Leonard. *The Dictionary of Vitamins: The Complete Guide to Vitamins and Vitamin Therapy.* New York: Thorsons Publishers, 1984.

Mindell, Earl. *Earl Mindell's New and Revised Vitamin Bible.* New York: Warner Books, 1985.

Mosby's Complete Drug Reference: Physicians GenRx. 7th ed. St. Louis, Mo.: Mosby Year Book, Inc., 1997.

Nutritional Labeling, How It Can Work for You. Bethesda, Md.: National Nutrition Consortium, 1975.

Pressman, Alan H., D.C., Ph.D., C.C.N., and Sheila Buff. *The Complete Idiot's Guide to Vitamins and Minerals.* New York: Alpha Books, 1997.

Silverman, Harold. *The Vitamin Book.* New York: Bantam Books, 1985.

Somer, Elizabeth, M.A., R.D., and Health Media of America. *The Essential Guide to Vitamins and Minerals.* New York: Harper Perennial, 1995.

Spoerke, David G., Jr. *Herbal Medications.* Santa Barbara, Calif.: Woodbridge Press Publishing Company, 1980.

Switzer, Larry. *Spirulina, the Whole Food Revolution.* New York: Bantam Books, 1982.

Time-Life Books. *The Drug & Natural Medicine Advisor.* Alexandria, Va.: Time-Life Inc., 1997.

Understanding Vitamins and Minerals. Emmaus, Pa.: Rodale Press, 1984.

United States Department of Agriculture. "Dietary Guidelines for Americans." Nutrition and Your Health. *Home and Garden Bulletin* No. 232 (1985).

United States Pharmacopeial Convention, Inc. *USP DI, Volume I, Drug Information for the Health Care Professional.* 17th ed. Taunton, Mass.: Rand McNally, 1997.

University of California at Berkeley Wellness Newsletter. New York: Health Letter Associates, 1984.

Willard, Mervyn D. *Nutrition for the Practicing Physician.* Menlo Park, Calif: Addison-Wesley Publishing Company, 1982.

Index

Note: Entries in **bold** refer to main headings

A

Absorption diseases, 117
Acid-base balance, regulates, 33, 59, 69
Acidophilus, 146–147
Adrenal glands, 156, 186
   aids in function of, 84
Alcoholism, 35, 59, 117
Algae. *See* Spirulina
Allergy symptoms, decreases, 147
Alphatocopherol. *See* Vitamin E
Alzheimer's disease, may treat, 87, 92, 162
Amino acids, 121–143
   aids metabolism of, 101
   defined, 121, 186
Anemia, 37, 39, 84, 101, 112
   defined, 186
   iron-deficiency, 48
   pernicious, 37, 87–88, 186
Anorexia nervosa, 37
Antacid, acts as, 29, 52
Antiaging remedy, 156
Antibodies, promotes production of, 128, 135
Anti-inflammatory, 160
Antioxidant, 54, 65, 74, 98, 126
Arginine, 122–123
Arsenic, 26–27
Arteriosclerosis, protects against, 169
Ascorbic Acid, 83–86
Astringent, natural, 160
Athletics, enhancing performance in, 155

B

B Vitamins, source of, 150
Bacteria, maintains balance, 146
Barley Grass. *See* Wheat Grass
Bee Pollen, 147–148
Beriberi, treats, 117
Beta-carotene. *See* Vitamin A
Bibliography, 194–195
Bile secretion, stimulates production of, 71
Bioflavonoids (Vitamin P), 148–149.
   See also Phytochemicals

Biotin (Vitamin H), 90–91
Bleeding disorders, treats, 109
Blood cells, promotes health of, 90
Blood-clotting,
   interferes with, 98
   regulates, 29, 109
Blood pressure
   maintains normal, 69
   reduces, 29, 67
Blood vessels, strengthens, 67
Blue-green algae. *See* Spirulina
Body fat, reduces, 153
Bone growth, promotes, 42, 52, 67, 80, 94
Bone health, promotes, 27, 29, 59, 109
Bone marrow, promotes health of, 48, 84, 90
Bones, broken, helps heal, 84
Boric acid, 28
Boron, 27–29
Brain, helps maintain normal function of, 112
Brewer's Yeast, 150–151
Bulimia, 37
Bulk. *See* Dietary Fiber
Burns, helps heal, 37, 39, 84, 117

C

Calcium, 29–32
Calcium absorption,
   helps control, 42, 67, 94
   increases, 27, 84
Calcium depletion, treats, 29
Cancer, protective against, 175
Carbohydrate metabolism, 54
Cardiovascular disease, reduces risk of, 67
Cartilage, 67, 151
Cautions when using supplements, 22–23
Cavities, prevents, 41, 42
Cell function, promotes, 45, 74, 126
Cell membrane, helps maintain, 28, 52, 92
Central-nervous-system function, 39
Chemotherapy, 124
Chloride, 33–34

INDEX